DEJA REVIEW™

Family Medicine

NOTICE

DEJA REVIEW™

Family Medicine

Mayra Perez, MD

Resident
Department of Family Medicine
The Methodist Hospital of Houston
Houston, Texas
Class of 2006
The University of Texas at Houston Medical School
Houston, Texas

Lindsay K. Botsford, MD

Resident
Department of Family Medicine
Baylor College of Medicine/Kelsey-Seybold Clinic
Houston, Texas
Class of 2007
Baylor College of Medicine
Houston, Texas

Winston Liaw, MD, MPH

Resident
Department of Family Medicine
Virginia Commonwealth University—Fairfax
Fairfax, Virginia
Class of 2006
Baylor College of Medicine
Houston, Texas
Class of 2005
Harvard School of Public Health
Boston, Massachusetts

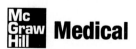

New York   Chicago   San Francisco   Lisbon   London   Madrid   Mexico City
Milan   New Delhi   San Juan   Seoul   Singapore   Sydney   Toronto

Deja Review™: Family Medicine

1 2 3 4 5 6 7 8 9 0   DOC/DOC   0 9 8 7

ISBN 978-0-07-148568-5
MHID 0-07-148568-6

This book was set in Palatino by International Typesetting and Composition.
The editors were Laura K. Wenham, Marsha S. Loeb, and Peter J. Boyle.
The production supervisor was Catherine Saggese.
Project management was provided by International Typesetting and Composition.
The text was designed by Marsha Cohen/Parallelogram.
RR Donnelley was printer and binder.

This book is printed on acid-free paper.

Library of Congress Cataloging-in-Publication Data

Perez, Mayra.
    Deja review : family medicine / Mayra Perez, Lindsay K. Botsford, Winston Liaw.
        p. ; cm. — (Deja review)
    Includes index.
    ISBN-13: 978-0-07-148568-5 (pbk. : alk. paper)
    ISBN-10: 0-07-148568-6
    1. Family medicine—Examinations, questions, etc.   I. Botsford, Lindsay K.   II. Liaw, Winston.   III. Title.   IV. Title: Family medicine.   V Series.
    [DNLM: 1. Family Practice—Examination Questions.
WB 18.2 P438d   2008]
    RC58.P445   2008
    610.76—dc22
                                              2007034081

To my mother and grandmother, for their incredible sacrifices; to John, for making my dreams come true; and to our little Julia, for existing perfectly.
—Mayra Perez

To my teachers and mentors who encouraged my curiosity and involvement in many pursuits; and to my family and friends who supported me throughout those adventures.
—Lindsay K. Botsford

To my parents and grandparents who encouraged me to never stop learning and supported me along the way; to my rocks: sis, who never ceases to inspire, and Eden, my instant happiness.
—Winston Liaw

Contents

Faculty Reviewer

Donald Briscoe, MD
Program Director
Methodist Hospital (Houston) Family
    Medicine Residency Program

Medical Director
Denver Harbor Clinic

Clinical Assistant Professor of Family
    Medicine in Medicine
Weill Medical College of Cornell University

Resident Reviewers

Ryan Buffington, MD
Chief Resident
Family Medicine Residency Program
The Methodist Hospital—Houston
Houston, Texas

Benjamin Mailloux, MD
Chief Resident
Department of Family Medicine
Virginia Commonwealth University—Fairfax
    Fairfax, Virginia

Student Reviewers

Mary Martha Bonar
Class of 2008
Ohio University College of Osteopathic
    Medicine
Athens, Ohio

Basim Khan
Class of 2008
David Geffen School of Medicine at UCLA
Los Angeles, California

Carrie Fathke
Class of 2007
University of Washington School of
    Medicine
Seattle, Washington

Contributing Authors

Lauren Sasha Blieden, MD
Resident
Department of Ophthalmology
Baylor College of Medicine
Houston, Texas
Class of 2007
Baylor College of Medicine
Houston, Texas

Chung-Yin Stanley Chan, MD
Resident
Department of Dermatology
Baylor College of Medicine
Houston, Texas
Class of 2007
Baylor College of Medicine
Houston, Texas

Lesley M. Crabbe, MD
Resident
Department of Internal Medicine
Barnes Jewish Hospital
Washington University
St. Louis, Missouri
Class of 2006
Baylor College of Medicine
Houston, Texas

Quynh-Thu N. Doan, MD
Resident
Department of Obstetrics and Gynecology
Baylor College of Medicine
Houston, Texas
Class of 2006
Baylor College of Medicine
Houston, Texas

Edgar I. Hernandez, MD
Resident
Department of Surgery
SUNY—Stony Brook University Medical
   Center
Stony Brook, New York
Class of 2006
The University of Texas—Houston Medical
   School
Houston, Texas

David Alvin Lee, MD
Resident
Department of Dermatology
The Johns Hopkins Hospital
Baltimore, Maryland
Class of 2006
Columbia University College of Physicians
   and Surgeons
New York, New York

Chalam Mulukutla, MD
Resident
Combined Internal Medicine and Pediatrics
   Program
Baylor College of Medicine
Houston, Texas
Class of 2005
Baylor College of Medicine
Houston, Texas

Stacey Rubin Rose, MD
Resident
Department of Internal Medicine
Baylor College of Medicine
Houston, Texas
Class of 2007
Baylor College of Medicine
Houston, Texas

Paulraj Samuel, MD, MPH
Resident
Department of Internal Medicine
University of Pittsburgh Medical Center
Pittsburgh, Pennsylvania
Class of 2006
Baylor College of Medicine
Houston, Texas
Class of 2005
Harvard School of Public Health
Boston, Massachusetts

Amy E. Schindler, MD
Resident
Department of Internal Medicine
Vanderbilt University Medical Center
Nashville, Tennessee
Class of 2006
University of Texas Southwestern Medical
    School
Dallas, Texas

Chirayu Shah, MD
Resident
Department of Internal Medicine
Baylor College of Medicine
Houston, Texas
Class of 2005
Baylor College of Medicine
Houston, Texas

Ruhi Singh, MD
Resident
Department of Ophthalmology
Baylor College of Medicine
Houston, Texas
Class of 2007
Baylor College of Medicine
Houston, Texas

Jennifer H. Tang, MD
Resident
Department of Obstetrics, Gynecology,
    and Reproductive Biology
Brigham and Women's Hospital
Massachusetts General Hospital
Boston, Massachusetts
Class of 2006
Baylor College of Medicine
Houston, Texas

Brian Tison, MD
Resident
Department of Pediatrics
Cincinnati Children's Hospital
Cincinnati, Ohio
Class of 2006
Baylor College of Medicine
Houston, Texas

Brian J. Williams
Class of 2008
Baylor College of Medicine
Houston, Texas

Justin E. Yanosik, MD
Resident
Department of Anesthesiology
Baylor College of Medicine
Houston, Texas
Class of 2007
Baylor College of Medicine
Houston, Texas

Preface

The format of this review book is intended for rapid-fire review, conducive to studying during five-minute breaks between patients or in the days leading up to your shelf exam. It is not intended to teach you everything about family medicine from scratch. You should already be familiar with the topics before using the quick-fire method. We recommend browsing the sections at the beginning of the rotation and identifying your strengths and weaknesses. It will give you a good idea of what subject areas to focus on with your preceptor during your rotation. As you become comfortable with certain topics, find the appropriate chapter and test your knowledge. We recommend reading the professional association summaries on hypertension (JNC7), hypercholesterolemia (ATP III), and diabetes (ADA Clinical Practice Recommendations) as early as you can during your rotation. We also recommend using the American Academy of Family Practitioners and United States Preventive Services Task Force websites as key family medicine references.

We value your feedback on this book. If sections are particularly helpful or inadequate, we would like to know. Send your comments, suggestions, or mnemonics to DejaReviewFM@gmail.com.

Acknowledgments

We would like to acknowledge Dr. Donald Briscoe for his hard work and support in helping make this book a success. His dedication to teaching inspires residents and students to continually improve their clinical knowledge and skills. We thank him for his example of professionalism and excellent patient care.

CHAPTER 1

Preventive Medicine

CANCER SCREENING

What is the United States Preventive Services Task Force (USPSTF)?

An expert panel that reviews literature and makes preventive care recommendations

How does the USPSTF grade its recommendations regarding which cancer screens should be routinely administered?

A = strongly recommends the service; *good evidence that benefit >> harm*

B = recommends the service; *at least fair evidence that benefit > harm*

C = no recommendation for or against the service; *at least fair evidence that the service improves health outcomes but benefit ≅ harm*

D = recommends *against* routine administration of the service to asymptomatic patients; *at least fair evidence that harm > benefit*

I = insufficient evidence for or against routine administration

EPIDEMIOLOGY

Explain the following descriptive (hypothesis forming) study designs.

Correlational

Uses population data such as comparing a country's alcohol intake to its prevalence of coronary artery disease

Case report

Descriptive study of factors that could be related to an outcome; uncontrolled

Cancer	Screen	Start age (years)	Frequency	USPSTF recommended grade for routine screening	Comments
Colorectal cancer The American Cancer Society (ACS) recommends the administration of 1 of these 5 protocols	1. Fecal occult blood test (FOBT) from 3 consecutive stool samples	50	Every year	A	
	2. Sigmoidoscopy	50	Every 5 years		
	3. FOBT + sigmoidoscopy	50	FOBT: every year; Sigmoidoscopy: every 5 years		FOBT + sigmoidoscopy is preferred to either one alone
	4. Double contrast barium enema	50	Every 5 years		
	5. Colonoscopy	50	Every 10 years		
Cervical cancer				A: sexually active with cervix D: >65 years old and not high risk* D: total hysterectomy for benign disease	

Cancer	Screening method	Age to begin	Frequency	USPSTF grade	ACS recommendations
	Pap smear = samples of squamous ectocervical (use the spatula) & columnar endocervical (use the cytobrush) epithelium; ↑dysplasia at the transition zone between the ectocervical and endocervical epithelium	3 years after the onset of sexual activity or 21 years old (whichever comes first)	Every year; at 30 years old women with three consecutive normal results may get screened every 3 years (except high-risk patients*)		
Breast cancer	Screening mammography ± clinical breast exam (CBE)	40	Every 1–2 years	B	USPSTF comments that the benefit is greatest for 50–65-years old women
Prostate cancer	Prostate specific antigen (PSA) and digital rectal exam (DRE)	50	Every year	I	PSA + DRE can detect early pathological changes but no studies have demonstrated ↓mortality

* High risk of cervical cancer = history of cervical cancer, exposure to diethylstilbestrol before birth, HIV, or immunocompromised

Cross-sectional	Assesses the outcome and exposure simultaneously
Can cross-sectional studies prove causality?	No. Because the temporal relationship between the variables is unknown

Give examples of the following analytic (hypothesis testing) study designs.

Observational	Cohort and case control studies
Interventional	Randomized controlled trials (RCTs)
How are patients in a case control study grouped and evaluated?	Persons with a known outcome (such as cancer) are identified as "cases" and those without the outcome as "controls." The study compares the groups, looking for multiple potential exposures of the outcome
How are patients in a cohort study grouped and evaluated?	Participants are divided into groups based on some common exposure (such as low-vs high-fat diets). The study compares multiple potential outcomes of the exposure
What are prospective studies?	At the study initiation, the disease has not occurred, and the study group is followed forward in time
What are retrospective studies?	At the study initiation, the disease has occurred, and the researcher looks back in time to identify potential etiologies

What is the term to describe the following?

The percent of the population with a disease at a given point in time (# persons with the disease / # persons in the total population)	Prevalence
The percent of the population who develop a disease over a period of time (# persons who develop the disease / # persons who are initially disease free in a population)?	Incidence

	Disease +	Disease −	
Exposure +	a	b	a+b = total exposed
Exposure −	c	d	c+d = total unexposed
	a+c = total with disease	b+d = total without disease	a+b+c+d = total persons

| What is relative risk? | The incidence of disease in the exposed compared to the incidence of disease in the unexposed |

| How do you calculate relative risk? | Relative risk = $[a/(a+b)]/[c/(c+d)]$ |

| When is relative risk used? | In cohort studies and RCTs |

| How do you calculate an odds ratio? | Odds ratio = $(a \times d) / (b \times c)$ |

| When is an odds ratio used? | In case control studies |

| Why are odds ratios used in case control studies? | In case control studies you cannot calculate disease development, so you cannot calculate relative risk. Odds ratios approximate the relative risk |

	Disease +	Disease −	
Test +	a = true positive (TP)	b = false positive (FP)	a+b = total with + tests
Test −	c = false negative (FN)	d = true negative (TN)	c+d = total with − tests
	a+c = total with disease	b+d = total without disease	a+b+c+d = total persons

| What does a "false negative" result mean? | A person with a disease who tests negative for that disease |

| What does a "false positive" result mean? | A person without a disease tests positive for that disease |

| Define sensitivity. | Percent of those with the disease that test positive |

| How do you calculate sensitivity? | TP/(TP+FN) = TP/(everyone with the disease) |

| Define specificity. | Percent of those without the disease that test negative |

| How do you calculate specificity? | TN/(TN+FP) = TN/(everyone without the disease) |

| What is more desirable in a screening test, high sensitivity or high specificity? | High sensitivity (*SnNOut*: In a sensitive [*Sn*] test, a negative result [*N*] helps to rule out [*Out*] disease) |

| What is more desirable in a confirmatory test, high sensitivity or high specificity? | High specificity (*SpPIn*: In a specific [*Sp*] test, a positive result [*P*] helps to rule in [*In*] disease) |

| What is positive predictive value (PPV)? | Percent of those with positive tests that actually have the disease |

How do you calculate PPV?	PPV = TP/(TP+FP) = TP/(all those with positive tests)
What is negative predictive value (NPV)?	Percent of those with negative tests that actually do not have the disease
How do you calculate NPV?	NPV = TN/(TN+FN) = TN/(all those with negative tests)
How does disease prevalence affect PPV and NPV?	Increasing prevalence leads to increasing PPV; Decreasing prevalence leads to increasing NPV

VACCINES IN ADULTS AND CHILDREN

What are examples of live vaccines?	Measles, mumps, and rubella (MMR); Sabin oral polio vaccine; Varicella-zoster virus (VZV)
Why is the oral polio vaccine no longer distributed in the United States?	Increased risk of vaccine-associated paralytic poliomyelitis
Which populations should avoid live vaccines?	Pregnant women; The immunocompromised; Close contacts of the immunocompromised
What are the standard childhood immunizations?	MMR; VZV; Hepatitis B; Hepatitis A; *Haemophilus influenzae* type b (Hib); Inactivated polio vaccine (IPV); Pneumococcal conjugate vaccine (PCV7); Diphtheria, tetanus, and acellular pertussis (DTaP)
What is the dosing schedule for the MMR vaccine?	Two doses: 12–15 months old and 4–6 years old
What is the dosing schedule for the VZV vaccine?	One dose: 12–18 months
What are the contraindications to the MMR, VZV, and IPV vaccines?	The Immunocompromised (except in asymptomatic HIV) and anaphylaxis to neomycin
Why should patients avoid salicylates for six weeks after VZV vaccine administration?	To prevent Reye's syndrome (fatal hepatoencephalopathy)
What is the dosing schedule for the hepatitis B vaccine?	Three doses: 0–1 month old, 1–4 months old, and 6–18 months old
What is the management of a child born to an HBsAg positive mom?	Give the first dose of the hepatitis B vaccine and hepatitis B immunoglobulin (HBIG) at birth

What is the dosing schedule for the hepatitis A vaccine?	Two doses: 1 year old and then 6–18 months later
What is the dosing schedule for DTaP?	Five doses: 2, 4, 6, and 15–18 months old, and 4–6 years old; give Td (tetanus and diphtheria toxoids) boosters every ten years
What is the dosing schedule for the Hib vaccine?	Four doses: 2, 4, 6, and 12–15 months old
Since the introduction of the Hib vaccine in 1987, the number of Hib (a cause of meningitis and epiglottitis) cases in children less than five years old has decreased by what percentage?	99%
What is the dosing schedule for the IPV?	Four doses: 2, 4, and 6 months old and 4–6 years old
What is the dosing schedule for PCV7?	Four doses: 2, 4, 6, and 12–15 months old
What is the dosing schedule for the meningococcal vaccine?	One dose: 11–55 years old
Who should be offered the meningococcal vaccine?	11–12 years old; Teenagers entering high school who were not previously vaccinated; College freshmen in dorms; Military recruits; Complement deficiency patients; Asplenic patients
Asplenic patients are particularly vulnerable to what kind of infections?	Encapsulated bacterial infections
What is the dosing schedule for the influenza vaccine?	Yearly (influenza has a high rate of mutation)
During which months should the influenza vaccine be administered?	Fall and winter months
Which patients should be offered the influenza vaccine?	Children 6–24 months old; Adults >50 years old; Patients with chronic respiratory disease, chronic kidney disease, diabetes, or cardiovascular disease; Health care workers; Nursing home residents; Pregnant women; Household contacts of high-risk patients
Which patients should not be offered the influenza vaccine?	Patients with anaphylaxis to eggs (since the vaccine is prepared from viruses grown in eggs)

When should the first dose of the human papillomavirus (HPV) vaccine be offered to females?	11–12 years of age
When should the second and third doses of the HPV vaccine be administered?	Second dose two months after the first and the third dose six months after the first
What age range of females should be offered the HPV vaccine?	9–26 years old
May females over the age of 26 years receive the vaccine?	Yes. However, studies are still ongoing to determine safety and efficacy in this age group
Why should females who have received the vaccine still be screened for cervical cancer?	The vaccine does not protect against all HPV types that cause cancer; Patients may not have received all the doses of the vaccine; Patients who already have acquired HPV may not get the vaccine's full benefit
Which patients should be offered PPV23?	Adults >65 years old; Patients with chronic respiratory disease, cardiovascular disease, diabetes, chronic liver disease, chronic renal failure, and nephrotic syndrome; Nursing home residents; The immunocompromised; Asplenic patients
What are the indications for revaccination with PPV23?	Patient received the vaccine ≥5 years previously and was <65 years old at the time of vaccination; Patient has chronic renal failure, asplenia, or is immunocompromised
Why can you not use PPV23 in children?	PPV23 contains polysaccharide antigens that are not immunogenic in children <2 years old (PCV7 contains seven capsular poly-saccharides conjugated to a protein)
Who should be given the herpes zoster (one dose) to prevent shingles and postherpetic neuralgia?	Adults >60 years old regardless of prior history of herpes zoster
Who should receive Tdap (a full dose of tetanus, reduced dose of diphtheria, and acellular pertussis)?	A single dose is recommended for adolescents 11–12 years old or in place of one Td booster in older adolescents and adults 19–64 years old

INFECTIVE ENDOCARDITIS PROPHYLAXIS

What is the theoretical basis for infective endocarditis (IE) prophylaxis?

Transient bacteremia (especially *Streptococcus viridans*) is common after invasive procedures

According to the American Heart Association's 2007 guidelines, prophylaxis is only recommended for which cardiac conditions?

Patients with prosthetic cardiac valves, previous infective endocarditis, congenital heart disease (CHD) in certain situations (unrepaired cyanotic CHD, repaired congenital heart defect with prosthetic material within the first six months post procedure, and repaired CHD with residual defects at the site of a prosthetic device); Cardiac transplantations who develop cardiac valvulopathy

Endocarditis prophylaxis is recommended for which dental procedures involving the above cardiac conditions?

All dental procedures that involve manipulation of gingival tissue or the periapical region of teeth or perforation of the oral mucosa

Which antibiotic regimens are recommended for dental procedures?

Able to take PO: amoxicillin; Unable to take PO: ampicillin, cefazolin, or ceftriaxone; Allergic to penicillins and able to take PO: cephalexin, clindamycin, azithromycin, or clarithromycin; Allergic to penicillins and unable to take PO: cefazolin, ceftriaxone, or clindamycin

Prophylaxis is recommended for which respiratory procedures involving the above cardiac conditions?

Procedures that involve incision or biopsy of the respiratory mucosa (e.g., tonsillectomy or drainage of an empyema)

Is prophylaxis recommended for bronchoscopy?

No. (Assuming that the respiratory mucosa is not biopsied)

Which antibiotic regimens are recommended for respiratory tract procedures?

The same regimens for dental procedures with the following caveat: if the infection is known or suspected to be caused by *Staphylococcus aureus*, then the regimen should contain an antistaphylococcal penicillin or cephalosporin or vancomycin (if unable to tolerate beta-lactams)

Is prophylaxis recommended for procedures on infected skin, skin structure, or musculoskeletal tissue involving the above cardiac conditions?

Yes

Which antibiotic regimens are recommended for procedures involving infected skin, skin structure, or musculoskeletal tissue?

The same regimens for dental procedures with the following caveat: for patients unable to tolerate beta-lactams or who are known to have a methicillin-resistant strain of staphylococcus, use clindamycin or vancomycin.

CHAPTER 2

Cardiology

HYPERTENSION

What is normal blood pressure (BP) in adults (units = mm Hg)?

Systolic blood pressure (SBP) <120 *and* diastolic blood pressure (DBP) <80

What is Prehypertension?

SBP of 120–139 *or* DBP of 80–89

Stage 1 hypertension (HTN)?

SBP of 140–159 *or* DBP of 90–99

Stage 2 HTN?

SBP ≥160 *or* DBP ≥100

List the five important causal factors for primary HTN.

1. Excessive weight
2. Sedentary lifestyle
3. Excessive sodium intake
4. Inadequate intake of fruits, vegetables, and potassium
5. Excessive alcohol intake

How do you diagnose HTN?

Two or more properly measured elevated BPs on each of two or more office visits

How should you position patients to take their BP?

After allowing them to sit for five minutes, legs supported, arm at level of heart

Fill in the blank: A BP cuff should encircle at least ___ of the patient's arm.

80%

In a patient with HTN, what review of systems questions should you ask about at each visit?

Chest pain; Shortness of breath; Abdominal pain; Headache, dizziness, blurry, and double vision

What is the most common symptom of HTN?

Typically no symptoms are reported

What are the goals of the history and physical examination for a HTN patient?

Assess lifestyle; Identify comorbidities; Assess overall cardiovascular disease (CVD) risk; Assess the extent of target organ damage; Rule out secondary causes of HTN

What physical examination components are especially important to document in patients with HTN?	Vital signs (including BP in both arms and body mass index [BMI]); Cardiopulmonary, neurologic, thyroid, and optic fundi examinations; Abdomen (aneurysm, organomegaly); Auscultation for renal, femoral, and carotid bruits; Extremities (pulses, edema)
Effectively controlling BP reduces patient morbidity and mortality by decreasing the incidence of what medical conditions?	CVD; Transient ischemic attack (TIA)/Cerebrovascular accident (CVA); Aneurysms; Dementia; Retinopathy; Chronic renal disease
BP control decreases the incidence of what specific cardiovascular diseases?	Heart failure; Left ventricular hypertrophy; Cardiomyopathy; Myocardial infarction (MI); Peripheral vascular disease (PVD)
True or false: The relationship between elevated BP and CVD is independent of other risk factors for CVD.	True
True or false: DBP is a more important CVD risk factor than SBP after the age of 50 years.	False. It's the opposite before 50
True or false: Beginning at a BP of 115/75, each incremental increase in BP of 20/10 doubles the risk of CVD.	True
What tests should be performed in patients with HTN before initiating therapy?	ECG; Blood glucose and hematocrit; Serum potassium and calcium; Creatinine (or calculated GFR); Fasting lipid profile; Urinalysis; Urine albumin excretion or albumin to creatinine ratio (optional)
How often should potassium and creatinine be checked thereafter?	Twice a year (base additional periodic labs on comorbidities)
What is the definition of albuminuria?	Greater than 300 mg of albumin excretion in urine over 24 hours
What is the definition of microalbuminuria?	30–300 mg albumin excretion in the urine over 24 hours
How do you measure albumin in the urine?	24-hour urine collection (gold standard) or spot albumin to creatinine ratio
What conditions warrant screening for micro/albuminuria annually?	Patients with HTN who also have diabetes or kidney disease
True or false: Renal function, as measured by the glomerular filtration rate (GFR),	False. It begins in the third or fourth decade; and by the sixth decade,

normally begins to deteriorate in the fifth or sixth decade of life.	GFR declines by 1–2 mL/min per year
True or false: Uncontrolled SBP can accelerate the decline of GFR by as much as 4–8 mL/min per year.	True
What is the definition of chronic kidney disease (CKD)?	Albuminuria or estimated GFR <60 mL/min/1.73 m^2
What is the most common cause of death in patients with CKD?	Stroke
What are the two most common causes of end-stage renal disease (ESRD)?	1. Diabetes 2. HTN
How often should patients with HTN see an ophthalmologist?	Once a year
Define the goal of BP management in patients without complicated HTN.	BP <140/90
Define the goal for BP management in patients with a treatment-altering comorbidity.	BP <130/80
Name these treatment-altering comorbidities.	CKD; Diabetes; or other CVD
True or false: Most people will reach their DBP goal when the SBP goal is achieved, so therapy should focus on lowering the SBP.	True
The term "prehypertension" is relatively new. Why is it important?	Patients in this category are at twice the risk of developing overt HTN than those with normal blood pressures
In the absence of comorbidities, are prehypertensive patients candidates for drug therapy?	No
What is the "therapy" for prehypertension?	Early intervention with healthy lifestyle modifications
Name lifestyle modifications for prehypertension and HTN.	1. DASH diet 2. Weight loss 3. Reduced alcohol intake 4. Regular aerobic exercise 5. Smoking cessation
What does DASH stand for?	Dietary Approaches to Stop Hypertension
Describe the DASH diet.	1. Rich in fruits, vegetables, and dairy products 2. Low in cholesterol and saturated and total fat

3. Rich in potassium and calcium
4. Less than 2.4 g (preferably 1.6 g) of sodium per day

True or false: Following the 1.6 g sodium DASH diet has similar effects to single-drug therapy.

True

Unless there is a compelling indication to start another medication, what drug should be initiated in cases of uncomplicated stage 1 HTN?

Low-dose thiazide diuretic

For the following compelling indications that may coexist with HTN, what medications should be used to lower BP (most patients require more than one medication)?

    Heart failure

Diuretic; Beta-blocker (BB); Angiotensin-converting enzyme inhibitor (ACEI); Angiotensin receptor blocker (ARB); Aldosterone antagonist

    Post-myocardial infarction

BB; ACEI; Aldosterone antagonist

    High risk of coronary artery disease

Diuretic; BB; ACEI; Calcium-channel blocker (CCB)

    Diabetes mellitus (Type I or II)

Diuretic; BB; ACEI; ARB; CCB

    Chronic kidney disease

ACEI or ARB in combination with a diuretic (may need loop diuretic)

    Recurrent stroke prevention

Diuretic; ACEI

What are the contraindications to BB use?

Severe reactive airway disease; Uncompensated heart failure; Severe peripheral arterial disease; Bradycardia or hypotension; High-grade AV block; or Sick sinus syndrome

When should you initiate treatment with *two* agents?

Patient's BP is >20/10 of the goal, even if current drug dosage is not maxed out.

About what percentage of HTN patients can have controlled BP on only one medication?

30%

After initiation of antihypertensive drug therapy, how often should patients follow up for medication adjustments?

Monthly, until BP goal is reached (more often if patient has Stage 2 HTN or comorbidities)

Once desired BP is achieved, how often should patients follow up?

Every 3–6 months

What is the diagnosis of a patient with DBP ranges between 90 mm Hg and 104 mm Hg in the health care provider's office, while remaining normal in all other settings?	"White Coat" hypertension
How can White Coat HTN be confirmed?	24-hour ambulatory BP cuff monitoring
When should ambulatory BP monitoring be considered?	Wide variation in self-reported BP readings; Evaluation of White Coat HTN; Assessment of drug effectiveness, side effects, or resistance
True or false: In-office BP readings better correlate with target organ damage than ambulatory BP readings.	False
What percent of patients have no direct identifiable cause of their HTN?	90–95%
What term is used to describe this type of HTN?	Primary (essential) hypertension
What percent of patients have secondary HTN?	5–10%
What is the most common cause of secondary HTN?	Renovascular hypertension
What processes cause renovascular HTN?	Atherosclerotic renal artery stenosis; Fibromuscular dysplasia; Vasculitis
Which is most common in older men?	Atherosclerotic renal artery stenosis
Younger women?	Fibromuscular dysplasia
For the following case scenarios, list the most likely cause of secondary HTN.	
Abdominal bruit on physical examination	Renovascular hypertension
Headache, sweating, and palpitations with periods of acute BP elevations	Pheochromocytoma
Diminished or delayed peripheral pulses, a bruit heard over the back, higher SBP in the upper extremities than in the lower extremities	Aortic coarctation
Truncal obesity, glucose intolerance, and abdominal striae	Cushing's syndrome
Therapy with ACEI or ARB precipitates acute renal failure	Bilateral renal artery stenosis

How do you evaluate the following causes of secondary HTN?

Sleep apnea	Sleep study with O_2 saturation
Drug-induced or drug-related HTN	Assesss for use of NSAIDS, Cyclooxygenase-2 (Cox-2) inhibitors, oral contraceptive pills (OCPs), steroids, and illicit drugs.
Primary aldosteronism (hypokalemia) or other mineralocorticoid excess state	24-hour urine aldosterone level or specific measurements of other mineralocorticoids
Renovascular disease	Doppler flow study or magnetic resonance (MR) angiography
Cushing's syndrome or other steroid excess	Dexamethasone suppression test
Pheochromocytoma	24-hour urinary catecholamines
Coarctation of the aorta	Computed tomography (CT) angiography
Thyroid or parathyroid disease	Thyroid stimulating hormone (TSH), and serum parathyroid hormone (PTH)

LIPID LOWERING

In healthy adults over 20 years of age, how often should lipid levels be checked?	Every five years
If hypercholesterolemia is identified, what further laboratory workup is indicated?	Fasting blood glucose; TSH; Liver function tests (LFTs); Creatinine
What is the primary target (lipoprotein) for cholesterol lowering therapy?	Low-density lipoprotein (LDL)
According to research, above what is LDL atherogenic?	Greater than 100 mg/dL
What determines the LDL cholesterol-lowering goal?	Risk of having a coronary heart disease (CHD) event sometime in the next ten years
List CHD risk factors.	Hypertension; HDL <40 mg/dL; Smoking; Male >45 years old; Female >55 years old; Family history of early CHD (first-degree male with CHD <55 years old; first-degree female with CHD <65 years old)

What high-density lipoprotein (HDL) level is considered a negative risk factor and may be counted as a minus one toward the overall number of CHD risk factors?

HDL >60

What lifestyle modifications can increase HDL?

Increase aerobic activity and moderate alcohol consumption (1–2 drinks per day)

List CHD equivalents.

1. Diabetes mellitus
2. Peripheral artery disease
3. Any combination of risk factors leading to cumulative 10-year CHD risk of over 20% (as determined by a risk calculator—widely available, including online)
4. Symptomatic carotid artery disease
5. Abdominal aortic aneurysm

Fill in the blank: Someone with known CHD or a CHD equivalent has a ___% risk of having another CHD event sometime in the next ten years.

Greater than 20

At what LDL level should lifestyle changes and medications be implemented?

See Table 2.1

What lifestyle modifications can lower LDL?

1. Dietary modifications
2. Increased physical activity
3. Smoking cessation
4. Weight loss

Table 2.1 LDL and Initiating Treatment

Category	LDL to start lifestyle change	LDL to consider drug therapy
CHD or risk equivalent	>100	>100 (< 100—optional goal)
2 risk factors, with 10 years risk 10–20%	>130	>130 (100–129—may consider tx)
2 risk factors, with 10 years risk <10%	>130	>160
0–1 risk factors	>160	>190 (160–189—may consider tx)

What dietary modifications should be made in regards to fat intake?

1. Total dietary fat should be less than 35% of total caloric intake (<10% polyunsaturated fat, <7% saturated fat, and minimal trans fat)
2. Cholesterol intake less than 200 mg/day

What is the LDL goal for patients with CHD or a CHD equivalent?

Less than 100

For patients with 0–1 risk factors and no CHD or a CHD equivalent, what is their LDL goal?

Less than 160

For patients with two or more risk factors and no CHD or a CHD equivalent, what is their LDL goal?

It depends if their ten-year CHD risk is <10%, 10–20%, or >20% (as determined by a risk calculator). See Table 2.2 or >20%

LDL <70 is an optional goal for which subset of patients?

Very high-risk patients (recent heart attack, metabolic syndrome, CVD with diabetes or severe or poorly controlled risk factors such as smoking)

What class of drugs represents the current first line pharmacotherapy in the lowering of LDL?

Statins

What is the mechanism of action of statins?

Inhibit HMG-CoA reductase

Statins may cause what potentially life-threatening side effect?

Rhabdomyolysis

What lab abnormality is possible with statins?

Elevations in aminotransferases (liver enzymes)

If a patient is on a statin, how often should you monitor liver enzymes?

6–12 weeks after initiation or dose change; then if they are normal, every 6–12 months thereafter

What drugs should be considered for the treatment of hypertriglyceridemia?

Fibric acid derivatives (Fibrates) and niacin

Table 2.2   LDL Goals

Category	LDL goal
CHD or risk equivalent (including 2 risk factors plus 10 years > 20% risk)	<100 (<70–optional goal)
2 risk factors, with 10 years risk 10–20%	<130 (<100-optional goal)
2 risk factors, with 10 years risk <10%	<130
0–1 risk factors	<160

How long after initial lifestyle modifications and/or medical therapy is started should lipids be rechecked?

Six weeks

HEART FAILURE

What is heart failure (HF)?

The heart's ability to pump is inadequate and unable to maintain the body's circulatory needs

What are the two types of heart failure?

Systolic dysfunction and diastolic dysfunction

Describe systolic dysfunction.

Dilated left ventricle with impaired ability to contract

Describe diastolic dysfunction.

Left ventricle appears normal but has impaired ability to relax and fill

What is a normal ejection fraction (EF)?

Greater than 55%

Which has a normal EF, systolic or diastolic HF?

Diastolic

Describe the role of anti-hypertensives in the treatment of HF.

Decrease afterload so the heart pumps against less resistance

How does chronic atrial fibrillation (AF) affect a patient with HF?

Tachycardia and the decreased atrial contraction worsens left ventricle (LV) filling, so AF rate control is important

What agents should be used to achieve AF rate control?

BB; CCB

What is BNP?

Brain natriuretic peptide—released from heart ventricle myocytes when they are stretched

What is a normal BNP level?

Less than 100

What is the BNP level seen in heart failure?

Greater than 500 (between 100–500 is inconclusive)

What are some common symptoms of left-sided HF?

Weakness and dyspnea with exertion (at rest in more advanced cases); Paroxysmal nocturnal dyspnea (PND); Orthopnea; Cough; Wheezing; Pink/Frothy sputum

What are some physical findings of left-sided HF?

Bilateral pulmonary crackles (rales); S3 gallop; Displaced PMI

What are some common symptoms of right-sided HF?

Abdominal pain and bloating; Nausea and vomiting; Anorexia; Constipation

What are some physical findings of right-sided HF?

Peripheral edema; Jugular venous distention (JVD); Hepatosplenomegaly; Hepatojugular reflux; Ascites

What are some common chest x-ray findings found in HF patients?

Pleural effusions; Pulmonary edema; Cephalization of pulmonary vessels; Cardiomegaly (cardiothoracic ratio >50%)

List cardiovascular diseases that lead to HF.

Ischemic heart disease; Hypertension; Valvular disease; Cardiac rhythm disorders; Cardiomyopathies

Describe the mechanisms by which ischemic heart disease may cause HF.

1. Chronic ischemia causes sub-optimal myocardial function
2. Previous MI leading to LV dysfunction and subsequent remodeling

What therapeutic strategies should be applied to HF patients with ischemic heart disease?

Medical treatment for angina; Direct efforts to modify cardiac risk factors; Consideration of surgery (stenting, angioplasty, coronary artery bypass grafting [CABG])

List the recommended lifestyle modifications for HF patients.

Dietary salt limitation; Exercise; Weight loss: Alcohol/Smoking cessation

What class of medication is used to treat fluid overload in both the acute and chronic setting?

Diuretics (usually loop diuretic such as furosemide)

For patients with HTN and HF what medications should be used to lower BP?

Diuretic; BB; ACEI; ARB; Aldosterone antagonist (spironolactone)

Which of these antihypertensives have shown some increase in patient survival?

BB (e.g. carvedilol and metoprolol suceinate); ACEI; ARB; Spironolactone

How have BBs and ACEIs specifically been shown to improve survival?

By reducing heart remodeling and decreasing sympathetic tone (less stress on heart)

What medications should be initiated for secondary prevention of further cardiovascular events?

Statin and aspirin

What additional medication combination may be of benefit to African American HF patients?

Hydralazine combined with nitrates

Describe the mechanism behind HF secondary to valvular disease.

Increased myocardial workload due to hemodynamic factors leads to myocardial dysfunction

What other general medical conditions may lead to HF?	Systemic lupus erythematous (SLE); Hemochromatosis; Sarcoidosis; Cocaine abuse; Alcohol abuse
What inflammatory disease is a significant cause of HF?	Myocarditis
List some causes of myocarditis.	Coxsackie B; Influenza; Adenovirus; Rheumatic fever (acute); HIV; Chagas' disease; Lyme disease
What lab findings may be abnormal in these patients?	Erythrocyte sedimentation rate (ESR) elevation; Creatine kinase (CK)/ troponin elevation during the acute phase; T-wave inversion or ST elevation on ECG
What are some common causes of acute exacerbations of HF?	Infection; Anemia; Acute myocardial infarction; Dietary indiscretions (high salt or water intake)
How do you manage new onset or acute exacerbation of HF requiring hospitalization?	Place patient on telemetry, give IV diuretics, monitor fluid balance and electrolytes closely, administer oxygen, control comorbidities (especially HTN), and evaluate precipitating causes of HF
How do you evaluate precipitating causes?	Echocardiogram; ECG; Chest x-ray (CXR); Blood tests
What blood tests should you order in the setting of acute onset of HF?	Complete blood count (CBC); Basic metabolic panel (BMP); Liver function tests (LFTs); Cardiac enzymes

CARDIOMYOPATHY

List the three types of cardiomyopathy.	1. Dilated cardiomyopathy (DCM) 2. Restrictive cardiomyopathy (RCM) 3. Hypertrophic cardiomyopathy (HCM)
Describe DCM.	May involve four-chamber dilation; typically involves at least LV dilation and systolic dysfunction
List some conditions that can lead to DCM.	Alcohol; Atrial flutter; Atrial fibrillation; Thyroid dysfunction; Pregnancy; Adenovirus; HIV; SLE; Cocaine; Beriberi (vitamin B_1 deficiency)
How is DCM evaluated?	Echocardiography

How is DCM treated?	It is treated as a systolic dysfunction.
Describe RCM.	Diastolic dysfunction without evidence of dilation or hypertrophy of the left ventricle
List some conditions that can lead to RCM.	Amyloidosis; Sarcoidosis; Glycogen storage diseases; Hemochromatosis; Idiopathic RCM
How is RCM evaluated?	Echocardiography (to reveal small ventricles and systolic abnormality in the presence of diastolic dysfunction)
How is RCM treated?	Similar to other disease states characterized by diastolic dysfunction
Describe HCM.	A cardiac sarcomere defect leading to hypertrophy of the ventricles
Is HCM typically inherited or acquired?	Inherited
What disease states fall under this general category?	Hypertrophic obstructive cardiomyopathy (HOCM); Asymmetric septal hypertrophy (ASH); Idiopathic hypertrophic subaortic stenosis (IHSS)
How is HCM evaluated?	ECG to demonstrate left axis deviation and left ventricular hypertrophy (LVH); and echocardiography to show ventricular thickening
How is HCM treated medically?	Calcium-channel blockers and BB given in high doses to act as a negative inotrope
When should surgical treatment (septal myomectomy) be considered?	When significant LV outflow tract obstruction is inadequately controlled by medical management

CORONARY ARTERY DISEASE

Describe the initial pathogenesis of atherosclerosis.	Endothelial injury leads to increased leukocyte adhesion to the endothelium, endothelial permeability, and endothelial release of hemostatic and vasoactive substances
How is angina pectoris diagnosed?	Clinical history of a retrosternal pressure-like or squeezing sensation, frequently with radiation to the arms or neck/jaw

What characterizes chronic stable angina?	Reproducibility with a consistent amount of exertion and long-standing symptoms
How is exercise-induced angina diagnosed?	Stress test demonstrates ST depression during exercise
Which stress-test findings may imply a poorer prognosis in cases of chronic stable angina?	ST depression greater than 2 mm; Ischemia at low stress levels; Hypotension resulting from exertion; Presence of ischemic changes in more than five ECG leads
What three general management strategies should be considered in chronic stable angina?	1. Modification of risk factors 2. Angina symptomatic relief via medication or interventional modalities 3. Treatment of other contributing diseases
What other diseases may exacerbate chronic stable angina?	Fever; Anemia; Congestive heart failure (CHF); Infection; Thyrotoxicosis
What medications may provide symptomatic relief of angina?	Nitrates; CCBs; BBs
Describe the mechanism by which nitrates provide symptomatic relief?	Vasodilation of . . . 1. Coronary vessels→ increases myocardial oxygen supply 2. Peripheral veins and arteries→ preload and afterload reduction→ decreases myocardial oxygen demand
On which do nitrates have predominate effect—veins or arteries?	Veins (and therefore preload)
Describe the mechanism by which BBs and CCBs provide symptomatic relief?	Decrease myocardial oxygen demand by decreasing heart rate, blood pressure, and contractility
If angina continues despite maximal medical management, what strategies may be employed?	Cardiac catherization to evaluate coronary anatomy; Revascularization can be considered via coronary angioplasty, stenting, or CABG
Describe Prinzmetal's variant angina.	Angina at rest characterized by transient coronary artery spasm and ST elevation
What conditions fall under the heading of acute coronary syndromes (ACS)?	Unstable angina (UA); ST-elevation MI (STEMI); Non-ST-elevation MI (NSTEMI)
What physical exam findings are typical of ACS?	Tachycardia; Transient S3 or S4; Hypertension; Mitral regurgitation

	secondary to ischemia of the papillary muscle
Describe UA.	New onset angina (less than two months) with only minimal exertion; Crescendo angina in the setting of existing stable angina; Angina at rest of greater than 20 minutes; Angina occurring greater than 24 hours post-MI
What ECG findings may be seen in UA?	ST depression or symmetric T-wave inversions
In what percentage of patients does UA progress to MI?	Approximately 5%
In cases of UA, what are the major steps for providing symptomatic relief and preserving myocardial function?	Provide analgesia; Improve coronary blood flow; Prevent coronary thrombosis; Decrease myocardial oxygen demand
What drug options should be considered to address analgesia?	Morphine to decrease pain and anxiety
Why is it important to control pain in a patient with UA?	Analgesia can decrease the sympathetic response (lower HR and BP) which decreases myocardial oxygen demand
When should antiplatelet therapy be started?	Immediately after UA is suspected
What drug options should be used to provide antiplatelet action acutely?	Aspirin 162–325 mg and clopidogrel 300 mg
What drug options should be used to provide long-term antiplatelet action?	Aspirin 81–325 mg and clopidogrel 75 mg, daily
What class of drugs should be used to control ischemia in all patients with UA/NSTEMI?	BB
Is thrombolytic therapy used in the treatment of UA and NSTEMI?	No
Following stabilization of the UA/NSTEMI patient, what further studies should be undertaken in low-risk patients?	Noninvasive stress testing
In intermediate-risk patients?	Noninvasive stress testing undertaken after stabilizing the patient with medications
In high-risk patients?	Cardiac catheterization followed by revascularization procedures if indicated

Define STEMI.	An acute coronary syndrome whereby a complete and persistent occlusion of a coronary artery takes place
What groups of patients are more likely to present with atypical symptoms of MI?	Women; Diabetics; The elderly
What accounts for most of the deaths that take place within a few hours of a STEMI?	Ventricular tachyarrhythmia
Describe the time-course of ECG changes in a STEMI.	See Table 2.3.
What does echocardiography show during STEMI?	LV hypokinesis or akinesis in the area supplied by the occluded vessel
What cardiac enzymes (biomarkers) are elevated in the setting of STEMI?	Troponin I; Creatine kinase-MB isoenzyme (CK-MB); Lactate dehydrogenase (LDH)
Which biomarker is the most sensitive and specific for myocardial injury?	Troponin
What two pharmacologic agents should be instituted immediately after the diagnosis of STEMI is made?	Aspirin and anti-thrombotic agents (unfractionated or low molecular weight [LMW] heparin)
Despite its increased effectiveness, when is _LMW_ heparin contraindicated?	Renal insufficiency
What further immediate steps should be taken?	MONA—**M**orphine, **O**xygen, **N**itroglycerin, **A**spirin; anxiolytics, BB
How should the first dose of aspirin be taken?	Chewed, to ensure rapid uptake
If the patient shows continued ST-elevation and has persistent angina, what therapy should be initiated?	Reperfusion with primary angioplasty or initiation of thrombolysis
Tissue plasminogen activator (tPA) can restore patency to an occluded coronary vessel in what percentage of patients?	Approximately 75–80%
Primary angioplasty can restore patency to an occluded coronary vessel in what percentage of patients?	Approximately 95%

Table 2.3 ECG Changes During a STEMI

Immediate	Minutes	Hours	24–48 hours	Day-weeks
Hyperacute T waves	ST elevation	Q-wave , T-wave inversion	ST back to baseline	T wave normalizes

Beyond what period of time from the onset of initial symptoms does thrombolysis lose effectiveness?	Six hours
What is the major limitation of primary angioplasty in this clinical setting?	Lack of widespread availability
Following thrombolysis, for how long should heparin be continued?	24–48 hours
How long should aspirin be continued?	Indefinitely
What other drugs should be initiated on a long-term basis?	BBs; ACEI; Statins
What diagnostic study should be performed several days after acute MI?	Echocardiography

VALVULAR HEART DISEASE

What are the physical findings in mitral valve regurgitation (MVR)?	Collapsing pulse and presence of a blowing holosystolic murmur
What might a patient with MVR complain of?	Fatigue; Dyspnea; Orthopnea
What is the medical therapy for MVR?	Angiotensin converting enzyme (ACE) inhibitors and digoxin
For patients with mitral valve prolapse, what medication can improve symptoms of palpitations and chest pain?	Low-dose BB
What is the clinically recognized sole cause of mitral stenosis (MS)?	Rheumatic fever
What physical findings are typically present?	Loud S1, opening snap, and low-pitched diastolic rumble during mid to late diastole
What is the mortality associated with non-surgically treated symptomatic MS?	58% mortality in ten years for patients with mild symptoms; 85% mortality in ten years for patients with mild to moderate symptoms
What medical therapy may be initiated for MS?	Diuretics for pulmonary edema; and rate control with digoxin or BBs
When should surgical referral for MS take place?	If experiencing moderate symptoms such as paroxysmal nocturnal dyspnea or hemoptysis
What are some of the causes of aortic insufficiency (AI)?	Aortic valvular dysfunction; Aortic aneurysm; Syphilis; Rheumatic disease

What are the signs and symptoms in AI?	Flushing; Sweating; Wide pulse pressure; Murmur
What murmur is characteristic of AI?	High-pitched soft blowing diastolic murmur at the left sternal border (ask patient to lean forward and hold their breath)
What medical therapy may be initiated for AI?	Digoxin or ACE inhibitors
Besides mitral regurgitation, what is the most common cause of valvular disease?	Aortic stenosis (AS)
What is a normal aortic valve area?	3–4 cm^2 in adults
What is the aortic valve area in critical AS?	Less than 0.8 cm^2
List the three most common causes of AS.	Bicuspid aortic valve; Degenerative changes associated with the aging process (primarily sclerosis); Rheumatic fever
What are the symptoms of AS?	Angina, CHF symptoms, Syncope
Describe common signs in aortic stenosis.	Normal to low blood pressure; "Parvus et tardus" (a weak and slow carotid pulse that often rises slowly and with a shudder); A crescendo-decrescendo murmur at the right second intercostal space that typically radiates to the neck
How should aortic stenosis be followed?	ECG and CXR annually to monitor for LVH and increased cardiac size
How should AS be treated if it is asymptomatic?	No intervention is indicated
How should the disease be managed once symptoms begin?	Surgery

CARDIOVASCULAR EXAMINATION

Name the diseases or abnormalities that first come to mind with the following cardiovascular physical examination findings.	
Laterally and/or inferiorly displaced PMI	Enlarged left ventricle, most often caused by HTN
Pericardial friction rub	Pericarditis

Split S2 during inspiration	None (this is a physiologic split S2)
Split S2 during expiration (paradoxical split)	Left bundle branch block (most common cause), aortic stenosis
Wide split S2 (that varies with respiration)	Pulmonic stenosis; Right bundle branch block; Mitral regurgitation
Fixed wide split S2 (not varying with respiration)	Atrial septal defect (ASD) or right ventricular failure
Narrow splitting of S2 (increased P2)	Pulmonary HTN
Physiologic S3	Children; Young adults, Pregnant women
Non-physiologic S3	CHF; Enlarged ventricles; Mitral or tricuspid regurgitation
Physiologic S4	Athletes
Non-physiologic S4	HTN; Coronary artery disease (CAD); Aortic stenosis
Continuous machine-like murmur (congenital)	Patent ductus arteriosus
Mid-systolic click with late systolic murmur	Mitral valve prolapse
Loud S1, opening snap, mid-diastolic rumble	Mitral valve stenosis
Bounding pulse, wide pulse pressure, and early diastolic murmur	Aortic regurgitation
Harsh systolic murmur, increased with Valsalva, often with S3 and S4	Hypertrophic cardiomyopathy
Decreased pulse pressure, paradoxical split S2, harsh ejection murmur radiating to carotids	Aortic stenosis
Holosystolic blowing murmur at the apex radiating to the axilla	Mitral regurgitation
Holosystolic blowing murmur at the lower left sternal border radiating to the sternum; inspiration increases intensity	Tricuspid regurgitation
Diminished P2 with widely split S2 (or inaudible P2 and thus no split), harsh mid-systolic murmur, most often found in children	Pulmonic stenosis
Harsh holosystolic murmur, very loud and often with thrill (congenital)	Ventral septal defect

HTN in the upper extremities with decreased pressure in the lower extremities, femoral pulse is slight or delayed, rib-notching on CXR	Coarctation of the aorta
Carotid bruit	Arteriosclerosis; Arterial aneurysm; Thyroid artery dilation; AV fistula

Describe the following findings of bacterial endocarditis.

Roth's spots	Retinal hemorrhages with white centers seen by fundoscopy
Splinter hemorrhages	Narrow and straight lines of hemorrhage underneath the finger and toenails
Janeway lesions	Non-tender, hemorrhagic macules, or nodules on the palms and soles
Osler nodes	Tender, red, raised lesions on the finger pads

What is pulsus paradoxus?	A patient's systolic BP falls more than 10 mm Hg (and causes weakening of the pulse) during inspiration.
What causes pulsus paradoxus?	Pericardial tamponade; Asthma; Shock; Pulmonary embolism
What is Beck's Triad of cardiac tamponade?	1. Jugular venous distension (JVD) 2. Hypotension 3. Muffled/distant heart sounds

CHAPTER 3

Hematology

ANEMIA IN ADULTS

What is anemia?	Reduced mass of circulating red blood cells (RBCs) (detected by reduced hemoglobin)
What are the typical signs and symptoms of anemia?	Dyspnea (at rest or exertional); Fatigue; Postural dizziness palpitations; Tachycardia; Conjunctival and skin pallor; High output congestive heart failure (CHF)
What specific vital signs should you take if you suspect hypovolemia?	Check blood pressure (BP) and heart rate supine, sitting, and standing (orthostatic vital signs)
Which group of patients does not become symptomatic until their anemia is severe?	Patients with chronic anemia
What is mean corpuscular volume (MCV)?	The average volume of RBCs
What is microcytosis?	RBCs are too small (MCV <80)
What are the three main causes of microcytic anemia?	1. Iron-deficiency anemia (IDA) 2. Anemia of chronic disease (ACD) 3. Thalassemia
What are the causes of IDA?	Too little iron in diet; Poor absorption of iron; Lead poisoning; Blood loss
What is the most common cause of IDA in men and postmenopausal women?	Gastrointestinal (GI) bleeding
What studies need to be done in a male with IDA?	A GI workup (upper endoscopy, colonoscopy, and small bowel imaging)
What studies need to be done in a postmenopausal female with IDA?	A GI workup and an endometrial biopsy
What is the most common cause of IDA in reproductive-age women?	Menometrorrhagia (heavy and irregular menses)

What is the treatment for IDA?
Treat the underlying blood loss and give ferrous sulfate supplement

How long should you give a ferrous sulfate supplement in order to adequately replenish iron stores?
Continue treatment for two months after the hemoglobin corrects itself.

In a person with IDA, effective iron supplementation should increase hemoglobin at what rate?
2–4 g/dL every three weeks

What is pica?
A craving for substances not fit as food (such as dirt, paper products, and ice)

Although rare, pica is a specific symptom of what type of anemia?
IDA

What is the treatment of pica?
It improves with treatment of IDA

What syndrome is associated with dysphagia and IDA?
Plummer-Vinson (rare, except in the world of pimping)

What is the triad that characterizes Plummer-Vinson syndrome?
1. Esophageal webs (causing dysphagia)
2. IDA
3. Atrophic glossitis

What is ACD?
Anemia associated with chronic infectious, inflammatory, or neoplastic disease

What is the treatment for ACD?
Treat the underlying disorder.

What lab work helps you distinguish between IDA and ACD?
Iron panel

Ferritin is an indicator of what?
Iron stores

What is transferrin?
An iron-transporting protein

What organ produces transferrin?
Liver

What is total iron-binding capacity (TIBC)?
An indirect measure of the amount of transferrin in the blood

How do you calculate percent TIBC saturation?
Serum iron divided by TIBC

What is a common iron panel profile for a patient with IDA?
Low ferritin (<40); High TIBC; Low percent TIBC saturation (<20%)

What is a common iron panel profile for a patient with ACD (clue: iron is present but not available for use)?
Normal or high ferritin; Low TIBC; Normal or low percent TIBC saturation

What is thalassemia?
Anemia caused by reduced alpha (alpha-thalassemia) and beta

(beta-thalassemia) globin protein production (hemoglobin = heme + globin)

Thalassemia is more common amongst which ethnic groups?
Asian; Mediterranean; African American

In a patient with thalassemia, what causes hepatosplenomegaly?
Extramedullary hematopoiesis

What lab test is used to diagnose thalassemia?
Hemoglobin electrophoresis

Even though thalassemia and IDA are both microcytic anemia, why is it important not to use iron to treat a patient with thalassemia?
Patients with thalassemia already have a chronic state of iron overload

What causes the chronic state of iron overload in thalassemia?
Increased GI iron absorption (secondary to accelerated iron turnover), multiple transfusions, or both

What is the treatment for thalassemia?
Transfusions and iron chelators

What is macrocytosis?
RBCs are too large (MCV >100)

What are the causes of macrocytosis?
Folate deficiency; Vitamin B_{12} deficiency; Certain drugs such as hydroxyurea and zidovudine (AZT); Increased lipid deposition (liver disease, hypothyroidism, hyperlipidemia); Alcohol abuse; Myelodysplastic disorders

How do folate and B_{12} deficiencies lead to the generation of large cells?
Interference with DNA synthesis leads to delayed nuclear maturation

Folate and vitamin B_{12} deficiencies produce what kind of cells on a peripheral smear?
Megaloblasts (immature RBCs) and/or hypersegmented neutrophils (at least five lobes)

How long does it take for folate deficiency to develop?
Months

Why?
Folate body stores (10,000 mcg) are small compared to the daily requirement (400 mcg)

What is the most common cause of folate deficiency?
Poor diet (classically associated with alcoholism)

What are other causes of folate deficiency?
Pregnancy/lactation (increase daily folate demand); Drugs that interfere with folic acid metabolism (trimethoprim, methotrexate, phenytoin)

What is the treatment of folic acid deficiency? | Folic acid 1 mg PO daily for 1–4 months

Deficiency of which vitamin, folate or B_{12}, causes neurological signs and symptoms and why? | Vitamin B_{12}; because it is needed for myelin synthesis

What specific neurological signs and symptoms may be seen with B_{12} deficiency? | Loss of vibration and position sense; Weakness; Spasticity; Ataxia; Dementia

What causes the loss of vibration and position sense? | Degeneration of dorsal column tracts

What causes the weakness and spasticity? | Degeneration of corticospinal (upper motor neuron) tracts

How long does it take for vitamin B_{12} deficiency to develop? | Years

Why? | B_{12} body stores (5000 mcg) greatly outweigh the daily requirement (9 mcg).

What foods contain B_{12}? | Meat and dairy products

Where is B_{12} absorbed? | Terminal ileus

What is the most common cause of vitamin B_{12} deficiency? | Pernicious anemia

What is pernicious anemia? | Impaired absorption of B_{12} secondary to antibodies to gastric intrinsic factor (IF)

What are the other causes of vitamin B_{12} deficiency? | Gastrectomy or terminal ileal resection; Blind loops (bacterial overgrowth competes for vitamin B_{12}); Pancreatic insufficiency (proteases free vitamin B_{12} prior to IF binding); Strict vegan diet

What are the treatment options for B_{12} deficiency? | Vitamin B_{12}, 1 mg IM daily for one week—then 1 mg weekly for four weeks; Vitamin B_{12}, 2 mg PO daily for four months; Vitamin B_{12} nasal spray (but comparative studies are lacking)

What are reticulocytes? | Immature RBCs that normally account for 1–2% of circulating RBCs

How can you determine whether or not the bone marrow is responding appropriately to anemia? | Check the reticulocyte index (RI)

How do you calculate the RI? | Percent reticulocytes x (actual hematocrit / ideal hematocrit)

What does an RI <2% indicate?	Decreased RBC production (bone marrow is not responding)
What does an RI >2% indicate?	Increased RBC production (bone marrow is responding appropriately to RBC loss or destruction)
What is the most common cause of normocytic (MCV = 80–100) anemia from decreased RBC production?	Anemia of chronic disease
What are other causes of normocytic anemia from decreased RBC production?	Malignant marrow invasion; Aplastic anemia; Chronic renal failure; Endocrine dysfunction (hypopituitarism, hypothyroidism)
What is aplastic anemia?	Failure of bone marrow to make all blood cell types (caused by injury to blood stem cells)
Which toxins cause non-idiopathic aplastic anemia?	Benzene; Arsenic, Chloramphenicol; Sulfas
How does chronic renal failure cause anemia?	Decreased erythropoietin production
What is erythropoietin?	A glycoprotein hormone, primarily made by the kidney, which regulates red blood cell production
What are the causes of normocytic anemia from increased RBC loss?	Acute blood loss; Hemolysis; Drugs (methyldopa, penicillin, and cephalosporins)
Which diseases cause RBC hemolysis?	Sickle cell; Hereditary spherocytosis; G6PD deficiency; Pyruvate kinase deficiency; Warm/cold-antibody hemolysis

VENOUS THROMBOEMBOLISM (DEEP VENOUS THROMBOSIS AND PULMONARY EMBOLISM)

What is Virchow's triad?	The three factors involved in thrombosis formation.
What are the three factors?	1. Stasis of blood flow 2. Vascular endothelial injury 3. Hypercoagulability
What is Homan's sign?	Calf pain with passive ankle dorsiflexion associated with the presence of a deep venous thrombosis ([DVT] a frequently pimped but unreliable examination finding)

What physical examination findings suggest a DVT?	Local edema (>3 cm diameter increase compared to the unaffected side); Pain; warmth; A palpable cord (indicating a thrombosed vein); Presence of newly developed varicose veins
What is the imaging study of choice to rule out DVT?	Compression ultrasonography
What is the role of D-dimers in the workup of suspected DVT?	D-dimer levels <500 ng/mL are helpful in excluding DVTs
What are the risk factors for thrombosis?	See Table 3.1
Do all DVT patients need a workup for an inherited thrombophilia?	No
What is the management of a DVT?	Unfractionated or low-molecular-weight heparin (LMWH) and warfarin
For how many days should treatment with heparin and warfarin overlap?	At least 4–5 days
If heparin and warfarin have overlapped sufficiently and international normalized ratio (INR) has been therapeutic for two consecutive days, what should you do?	Discontinue heparin and continue warfarin alone.
How long should you continue oral anticoagulation with warfarin in the following scenarios?	
The cause of the venous thromboembolism (VTE) is reversible	Three months
It is the patient's first idiopathic VTE	6–12 months
The cause of the VTE is irreversible or if the patient has cancer	Indefinitely
What does INR stand for?	International normalized ratio
By whom and why was it developed?	By the World Health Organization (WHO) in order to standardize prothrombin times
What INR is considered therapeutic for warfarin treatment of DVTs?	2–3
What should be done if anticoagulation is contraindicated (e.g., active bleeding) or if anticoagulation has failed?	Place an Inferior Vena Cava (IVC) filter.
Is LMWH at least as effective as unfractionated heparin?	Yes

Table 3.1   Inherited and Acquired Risk Factors for Thrombosis

	Risk factor	Mechanism /Comments
Inherited	Protein **C** (PC) deficiency	PC inactivates coagulation factors (CF) 5a and 8a
Remember **CLOTS**	Factor 5 **L**eiden mutation	• With the mutation, factor 5 is resistant to protein C inactivation • The most common inherited cause
	Pr**O**thrombin (aka CF 2) gene mutation	The mutation increases CF 2 synthesis
	Anti**T**hrombin deficiency	
	Protein **S** (PS) deficiency	The action of PC is dependent on PS
Acquired	Malignancy	• Increased production of procoagulants • Check stool for occult blood (colorectal cancer) • Rectal exam in males (prostate cancer) • Pelvic exam in females
	Trauma	
	Pregnancy	Increased stasis from uterine obstruction of venous return and increased PC resistance
	Drugs	e.g., oral contraceptive pills, hormone replacement therapy, and tamoxifen
	Immobilization	
	Heart failure	
	Hyperhomocysteinemia	
	Antiphospholipid antibodies	• *In vitro* increase in aPTT that does not correct with mixing • Ask about prior fetal loss • Ask about meds (hydralazine, procainamide, and phenothiazines)
	Myeloproliferative disorders	i.e., essential thrombocythemia and polycythemia vera
	Hyperviscosity syndromes	i.e., Waldenstrom's macroglobulinemia and multiple myeloma
	Recent surgery	Especially orthopedic surgeries
	Nephrotic syndrome	Loss of antithrombin, PC, and PS
	Obesity	
	Prior venous thromboembolism	

What are the advantages of using LMWH versus unfractionated heparin?

Longer half-life allows for once or twice daily dosing; Doses are fixed; Monitoring of the activated partial thromboplastin time (aPTT) is not required; Thrombocytopenia is less likely

What percentage of symptomatic, untreated, proximal DVT patients will develop pulmonary embolism?

50%

What are the symptoms associated with pulmonary embolism (PE)?

Dyspnea; Pleuritic pain; Cough; Hemoptysis

What are the signs associated with PE?

Tachypnea; Rales; Diaphoresis; Tachycardia; Heart gallop; A loud second heart sound

What chest x-ray (CXR) findings suggest a PE?

Atelectasis; Hampton's hump; Westermark's sign

What is Hampton's hump on CXR?

A triangular pleural-based density with an apex that points toward the hilum

What is Westermark's sign?

Oligemia distal to the infarction

Although the ECG is often normal, a PE may cause what ECG changes?

Sinus tachycardia; Right bundle branch block; $S_I Q_{III} T_{III}$

What is $S_I Q_{III} T_{III}$?

Prominent S wave in lead I; Q wave in III; T-wave inversion in III

What arterial blood gas findings suggest PE?

Hypoxemia; Hypocapnia; Respiratory alkalosis

What other diagnostic studies are used in suspected PE?

D-dimer; Ventilation/perfusion (V/Q) scan; Spiral CT; Pulmonary angiography

CHAPTER 4

Gastroenterology

INFECTIOUS DIARRHEA

What factors in a patient's history suggest that diarrhea is infectious in etiology?

Ingestion of raw food, seafood, or picnic food; Recent travel (foreign or camping); Hospitalization, nursing home care, or day care; Anal intercourse; IV drug use; Sick contacts

What time course of a patient's diarrhea usually reflects an infectious etiology?

Acute diarrhea, with duration less than two weeks

What are the major bacterial causes of diarrhea?

Salmonella; Shigella; Staphylococcus aureus; Campylobacter; Escherichia coli; Yersinia enterocolitica; Vibrio parahaemolyticus; Vibrio cholerae; Bacillus cereus; Clostridium difficile

What are the major viral causes of diarrhea?

Rotavirus and caliciviruses (such as Norwalk virus)

What are the major parasitic causes of diarrhea?

Giardia; Entamoeba histolytica; Cryptosporidium

What is the most common cause of pediatric infectious diarrhea?

Rotavirus

What is the mechanism of transmission of rotavirus?

Fecal-oral

In what season is rotavirus most common?

Winter

What is the usual etiologic agent of "traveler's diarrhea"?

Bacteria such as enterotoxigenic *E. coli*

How can travelers reduce their risk of developing diarrhea?

Avoid tap water, fruits, salads, uncooked or under-cooked foods, and other foods that may be contaminated; Use of antibiotic prophylaxis is controversial

What is dysentery?

Bloody diarrhea containing mucus and polymorphonuclear leukocytes

	(inflammation of the colonic or ileal mucosa by invasion of organisms or toxin-induced injury)
What organisms cause dysentery?	*Campylobacter; Salmonella; Shigella; E. coli* O157:H7
True or false: Most cases of acute diarrhea are infectious and self-limited in nature.	True
How is acute diarrhea generally treated?	Patients without signs of systemic toxicity may be treated symptomatically (antidiarrheals such as loperamide or bismuth subsalicylate) and with oral fluid and electrolyte replacement
How should you manage patients with bloody diarrhea, high fever, or signs of systemic toxicity?	Avoid antimotility agents; Order stool studies (fecal leukocytes, bacterial culture, *C. difficile* toxin, and ova and parasites); Start antibiotics
What is hemolytic uremic syndrome (HUS)?	Dysentery; Renal failure; Microangiopathic hemolytic anemia; Thrombocytopenia
What causes it?	A Shiga-like toxin produced by the *E. coli* O157:H7 strain, which has been linked to contaminated foods (animal feces)
What patient populations are typically affected?	Children and elderly
How is it treated?	Supportive measures. Avoid antibiotics and antimotility agents (use in HUS has been associated with increased morbidity and mortality)
What pathogen causes pseudomembranous colitis?	*C. difficile*
When is the intestinal tract most susceptible to overcolonization with *C. difficile*?	After alteration of normal gut flora by antibiotics or chemotherapy
What does *C. difficile* toxin cause?	Secretory or bloody diarrhea and an inflammatory response
How is it typically diagnosed?	Identification of *C. difficile* toxin in stool and pseudomembranes on colonoscopy
How is it treated?	Cessation of implicated antibiotic. Metronidazole is the drug of choice for treatment, but vancomycin given orally is an alternative

HEPATITIS B

How is Hepatitis B virus (HBV) transmitted?	Through infected blood, saliva, vaginal secretions, and semen
What percent of those infected with HBV will develop chronic liver disease?	10%
Which virological marker is the first to emerge after infection with HBV?	Hepatitis B surface antigen (HBsAg)
Which virological marker correlates with the infectivity of HBV?	Hepatitis B e antigen (HBeAg)
Which virological marker allows you to distinguish between recent and chronic infection with HBV?	Hepatitis B core antibody (HBcAb)
If HBcAb IgM is positive?	Recent infection
If HBcAb IgG is positive?	Chronic infection
Interpret these Hepatitis B virological marker panels.	
HBsAg negative, anti-HBsAb positive, and anti-HBc IgG	Past HBV exposure
HBsAg negative and anti-HBsAb positive	Prior immunization
HBsAg positive, anti-HBsAb negative, and anti-HBc IgM	Acute hepatitis
HBsAg positive and anti-HBc IgG	Chronic hepatitis
How does an acute infection with HBV present?	Viral prodrome 4–12 weeks after infection; then with jaundice, scleral icterus, enlarged liver, and right upper quadrant pain
Which laboratory tests may appear elevated during acute infection with HBV?	Aspartate transaminase (AST); Alanine transaminase (ALT); Bilirubin; Alkaline phosphatase; Lymphocytes (especially atypical); Prothrombin time (PT)

GASTROESOPHAGEAL REFLUX DISEASE

What is gastroesophageal reflux disease (GERD)?	Pathologic reflux of acidic contents from the stomach into the esophagus causing symptoms or complications

What is physiologic reflux?	Reflux occurring after eating, for only short periods of time, and causing no symptoms
What is reflux esophagitis?	A subset of GERD cases that have evidence of esophageal inflammation on endoscopy or biopsy
What pathophysiologic factors may contribute to GERD?	Decreased resting amplitude of the lower esophageal sphincter; Impaired clearance of acid from the esophagus; Decreased mucosal protective mechanisms
What symptoms do patients with GERD typically complain of?	Heartburn; Regurgitation of acidic material; Dysphagia
When do symptoms of GERD typical occur?	After meals and when lying in recumbent position
What are some atypical symptoms of GERD?	Chest pain; Water brash (hypersalivation); Odynophagia; Nausea; Asthma; Laryngitis; Cough
What is the differential diagnosis of GERD?	Esophageal motility disorders; Infectious esophagitis; Pill esophagitis; Coronary artery disease; Gastritis; Peptic ulcer disease; Non-ulcer dyspepsia; Biliary tract disease
How are most cases of GERD diagnosed?	From the patient's history and a therapeutic response to an anti-reflux regimen of lifestyle and dietary modifications and/or acid suppression medication
When should you consider including endoscopy in your diagnostic workup?	The patient has odynophagia; Dysphagia; Weight loss; Early satiety; Bleeding or symptoms refractory to treatment.
In regards to 24-hour ambulatory esophageal pH:	
What patients are good candidates?	Those not responding to empiric medication and don't show evidence of inflammation on endoscopy
What can the test help demonstrate?	It can confirm the presence of reflux and the association of symptoms to episodes of reflux
What are the complications of GERD?	Esophagitis; Esophageal ulcers; Strictures; Barrett's esophagus;

	Iron-deficiency anemia; Extraesophageal manifestations such as asthma, cough, and laryngitis
What is Barrett's esophagus?	Metaplasia from squamous to columnar epithelium in the lower esophagus, resulting from chronic reflux
When should endoscopic surveillance for Barrett's esophagus be considered?	When symptoms have existed for over five years
Barrett's esophagus puts patients at increased risk for what malignancy?	Adenocarcinoma of the esophagus, which occurs in 10% of Barrett's esophagus cases
Name the available treatment/management for GERD under the following categories. (Note: Remember that the therapy must be titrated to the severity of the symptoms)	
Dietary modifications	Avoiding large meals; Not eating for 2–3 hours prior to reclining; Avoiding chocolate, cola, alcohol, coffee, and fatty food intake
Lifestyle modifications	Elevating the head of the bed; Weight loss (if obese); Smoking cessation
Avoidance of medications that may contribute to reflux	Oral bisphosphonates; Calcium-channel blockers; Anticholinergics; Sedatives; Theophylline
Drug therapy to reduce acid	Antacids; H2-blockers; Proton pump inhibitors (PPI)
What are the indications for anti-reflux surgery (Nissen fundoplication, etc.)?	Persistent or recurrent symptoms refractory to medical management; Severe esophagitis; Barrett's esophagus; Stricture; Recurrent aspiration or pneumonia associated with GERD

PEPTIC ULCER DISEASE

What are the two major etiologies of peptic ulcer disease (PUD)?	*Helicobacter pylori* (*H. pylori*) infection and nonsteroidal anti-inflammatory drug (NSAID) use
What symptoms do patients with PUD have?	Epigastric pain of a burning or gnawing quality that may radiate to the back

Describe the typical pain associated with:

Duodenal ulcers	Pain is relieved by food intake or antacids, but recurs 2–3 hours after meals and during the night on an empty stomach
Gastric ulcers	Pain occurs very soon after meals and is less responsive to antacids

What are the complications of peptic ulcers?

Perforation; Penetration; Hemorrhage; Pyloric outlet obstruction

How does perforation present?

Sudden onset of diffuse and severe abdominal pain

How does hemorrhage present?

Hematemesis; Melena; Nausea; Dizziness

How does pyloric outlet obstruction present?

Nausea and vomiting

What is the differential diagnosis of PUD?

Non-ulcer dyspepsia (functional dyspepsia); Drug-induced dyspepsia; Gastric carcinoma; Duodenal neoplasia; Crohn's disease; Granulomatous disease; Gastric infections; Duodenal infections

How is PUD diagnosed?

The clinical history raises suspicion for PUD, and confirmation can be made by upper endoscopy or a radiographic upper gastrointestinal (GI) series.

How is a peptic ulcer diagnosed by upper GI series?

Barium in a round or oval ulcer crater

How do the following differ in appearance on an upper GI series?

Benign gastric ulcer	Smooth and symmetric mucosal folds radiating to the edge of the crater or to a smooth edematous ring
Gastric cancer	An ulcer within a mass protruding into the gastric lumen; Irregular filling defects in the ulcer crater; Irregularity of the mucosal folds approaching the margin of the crater

Why must gastric ulcers be biopsied on endoscopy?

To detect malignancy

What is *H. pylori*?

A spiral, gram-negative urease-producing bacillus

H. pylori infection increases the risk of what malignancies?	Gastric adenocarcinoma and mucosa-associated lymphoid tissue (MALT) lymphoma, which frequently regresses with *H. pylori* eradication
What noninvasive tests are available to test patients for *H. pylori* infection?	Serum *H. pylori* IgG antibody serology; Carbon-labeled urea breath testing; Stool antigen testing
Invasive tests	A rapid urease assay (CLO test) and histopathologic examination of biopsy specimens are available for patients undergoing upper endoscopy

In regards to the medical treatment of peptic ulcers:

What is the standard of care?	Testing for and eradicating *H. pylori*, and acid suppression
How is acid suppression achieved?	PPI or an H2-blocker
What exposures should the patient avoid?	Foods that reproduce dyspepsia; Cigarette smoking; NSAIDs and aspirin if possible
How is *H. pylori* infection eradicated?	PPI for acid suppression and antibiotics twice daily for 10–14 days (clarithromycin, and amoxicillin or metronidazole)
When should PUD be managed surgically?	Peptic ulcers refractory to medical therapy; Recurrent peptic ulcers; Ulcer disease that is complicated by hemorrhage, penetration, perforation, or obstruction; Duodenal ulcers >5 cm in size
What is the basic goal of peptic ulcer surgery?	Selective vagotomy to denervate the acid-secreting parietal cells of the stomach
What is Zollinger-Ellison syndrome?	Hypersecretion of gastric acid caused by a gastrin-secreting islet cell tumor of the pancreas, resulting in multiple peptic ulcers that may be in unusual locations and are refractory to standard medical treatment or recurrent after surgery

GALLSTONE DISEASE

True or false: Calcium gallstones are the most common type.	False. 80% are cholesterol stones

What risk factors exist for gallstones?

Age >40 years; Female gender; Pregnancy; Oral contraceptive or estrogen replacement therapy; Obesity; Rapid weight loss; Native American ethnicity; Family history of first-degree relatives with gallstones

What is biliary colic?

Recurrent pain attacks that result from the gallbladder contracting against a gallstone in the gallbladder outlet

Where is the pain typically located?

In the right upper quadrant or epigastric region

Where does the pain classically radiate?

To the back or right shoulder

What is its relationship to food intake?

The pain classically follows a fatty meal by about an hour, progresses to a constant plateau that lasts over an hour, and then subsides over the next few hours

True or false: Patients with biliary colic exhibit fever, tachycardia, and peritoneal signs.

False. But the patient may exhibit voluntary guarding

What is the most widely used test in diagnosing gallstones?

Ultrasonography

How does a gallstone appear on ultrasound?

An echogenic focus that casts an acoustic shadow and is gravitationally dependent

Can gallstones be seen on plain abdominal x-ray?

Rarely

Why?

Only 10% of gallstones have enough calcium to be radiopaque

In patients with a typical history of biliary colic but no evidence of gallstones on ultrasound, what other diagnostic tools can be used?

Bile microscopy; Endoscopic ultrasound; CT of the abdomen; HIDA scan

How should patients with biliary colic and gallstones evidenced on ultrasound be treated?

Pain control for acute biliary colic, using either meperidine or NSAIDs, until definitive treatment of cholecystectomy can be carried out

Why is meperidine preferred over morphine in patients with biliary symptoms?

It causes less Sphincter of Oddi spasm

Why should patients with biliary colic have a cholecystectomy?

To definitively remove stones and prevent future attacks and complications such as cholecystitis

In patients with biliary colic and gallstones evidenced on ultrasound who are not good surgical candidates, what are some other treatment modalities?

Oral dissolution therapy with bile acids (but this may take up to two years!); Chemical lavage of the gallbladder; Shock wave lithotripsy. All of these nonsurgical modalities are rarely used

Should patients who are asymptomatic but have gallstones incidentally discovered on ultrasound undergo cholecystectomy?

No

Why?

The risk of surgical complications is greater than the risk of developing symptoms or complications of gallstones

Are there exceptions?

Yes. Patients at increased risk of gallbladder cancer (e.g., Native Americans, porcelain gallbladder, gallbladder adenomas); Patients with hereditary spherocytosis or sickle cell disease; Morbidly obese patients undergoing gastric bypass surgery

What are the complications of gallstones?

Acute cholecystitis; Ascending cholangitis; Acute biliary pancreatitis; Gallstone ileus; Gallbladder cancer

What are the typical symptoms of acute cholecystitis?

Severe right upper quadrant (RUQ) or midepigastric pain, radiating to the back or shoulder, in association with nausea and/or vomiting and anorexia

What are the key physical examination findings in acute cholecystitis?

Fever; Tachycardia; RUQ tenderness; Peritoneal signs; Positive Murphy's sign

What is a positive Murphy's sign?

Patient's inspiratory arrest caused by severe pain when asked to inspire deeply as the examiner palpates in the area of the gallbladder

What are the key lab findings of acute cholecystitis?

Leukocytosis with a left shift

What ultrasound findings support a diagnosis of acute cholecystitis?

The presence of gallstones; Gallbladder wall thickening; Pericholecystic fluid; A sonographic Murphy's sign

What test can be used to diagnose acute cholecystitis if the ultrasound was inconclusive?

HIDA scan

How should acute cholecystitis be treated?	IV fluids; NPO status; Pain control with opioids or ketorolac; Empiric antibiotics; Cholecystectomy
Describe acalculous cholecystitis.	Cholecystitis developing without the presence of gallstones (5–10% or cases of acute cholecystitis)
Acalculous cholecystitis usually occurs in what type of patients?	Critically ill patients or following major surgery or trauma, often in the setting of total parenteral nutrition (TPN)
What is Charcot's triad?	1. Fever 2. Jaundice 3. RUQ pain This triael signals ascending cholangitis
How does cholangitis develop?	From stasis and infection of the biliary tract, usually due to obstruction of the common bile duct by a stone
What is Reynold's pentad?	1. Altered mental status 2. Hypotension 3. Fever 4. Jaundice 5. RUQ pain
When does Reynold's pentad occur?	Suppurative cholangitis (associated with significant morbidity)
What lab findings are consistent with ascending cholangitis?	Leukocytosis with left shift; Elevated alkaline phosphatase; Gamma-glutamyl transpeptidase (GGT); Conjugated bilirubin
What imaging study is indicated for ascending cholangitis?	Ultrasound (looks for common bile duct dilation and gallstones)
How are patients with ascending cholangitis treated initially?	NPO, IV hydration, and empiric broad-spectrum antibiotics to cover gram-negatives and enterococcus
Under what circumstances is urgent biliary drainage required?	Hypotension; Mental confusion; Fever >102
In what percentage of patients with gallstones does biliary pancreatitis develop?	5%
What percentage of acute pancreatitis is caused by gallstones?	33%
What is gallstone ileus?	Mechanical bowel obstruction caused by a gallstone that has passed

through a biliary-enteric fistula and become impacted in the ileum

In what patient population is gallstone ileus most common?

Elderly patients

DIVERTICULAR DISEASE

What are diverticula?

Sac-like protrusions of the colon wall

What is the difference between diverticulosis and diverticulitis?

Diverticulosis describes the presence of diverticula, while diverticulitis is inflammation of those diverticula.

What is the prevalence of diverticular disease?

Less than 5% at age 40 to 65% at age 85

Of individuals with diverticulosis, what percent:

    Are asymptomatic

70%

    Develop diverticulitis

20%

    Develop diverticular bleeding

10%

Are the diverticula in diverticulosis "true" or "false?"

False. They don't contain all the layers of the colonic wall (mucosa and submucosa herniate through the muscle layer and are covered only by serosa)

Where do diverticula develop?

At points of weakness, where the vasa recta penetrates the circular muscle layer

What is thought to cause diverticula?

Increased colon pressure by enhanced peristaltic contractions and a low-fiber diet

Where in the colon do patients tend to get diverticula?

95% have sigmoid diverticula, while 35% also have disease proximal to the sigmoid

What causes diverticulitis?

Micro-perforation of diverticula by increased intraluminal pressure or inspissated food particles, resulting in inflammation and focal necrosis

What symptoms does diverticulitis cause?

Left lower quadrant (LLQ) pain, with or without nausea and vomiting; Constipation; Diarrhea; Irritative urinary symptoms

How does diverticulitis present on physical examination?	LLQ tenderness, with or without abdominal distention; Tender palpable mass; Low-grade fever
What are the key lab findings in diverticulitis?	
White blood cell count	Mild leukocytosis (but a normal white count does not exclude the diagnosis)
LFTs and amylase	Normal (amylase may be elevated if there is perforation with peritonitis)
Urine analysis/culture	Sterile pyuria (but colonic flora on urinary culture suggest a colovesical fistula)
What are the key CT findings in diverticulitis?	Increased soft tissue density within pericolic fat; Colonic diverticula; Bowel wall thickening
What are the complications of diverticulitis?	Abscess; Peritonitis; Fistula; Obstruction (these are all identifiable by CT)
How should you treat and/or manage the following?	
Uncomplicated acute diverticulitis	Bowel rest; IV hydration; Antibiotics (cover gram-negative rods and anaerobes). No colonoscopy in acute phase secondary to risk of perforation
Follow-up of uncomplicated acute diverticulitis	Colonoscopy or flexible sigmoidoscopy plus barium enema 2–6 weeks after resolution to rule out cancer and determine extent of disease
How should you treat and/or manage the following complications of diverticulitis?	
Perforation plus peritonitis	Emergency resuscitation; Broad-spectrum IV antibiotics; Emergency surgical exploration
Obstruction	Surgical exploration to differentiate from carcinoma
Abscess	Often can be drained by CT guidance, but surgical intervention may still be necessary
What causes diverticular bleeding?	A penetrating arterial vessel becomes draped over a diverticulum as it forms (with only mucosa separating the vessel from the lumen) so when

weakened over time, the vasa recta rupture into the lumen

True or false: Diverticular bleeding is painful but usually self-limited.

False. It is painless, however, it is usually self-limited

What dietary recommendations are made for patients with diverticular disease?

High-fiber diet

INFLAMMATORY BOWEL DISEASE

What two diseases are classified as inflammatory bowel disease (IBD)?

Ulcerative colitis (UC) and Crohn's disease

What layer(s) of the colon wall are inflamed in UC?

Mucosal layer only

What layer(s) of the colon wall are inflamed in Crohn's disease?

All layers (transmural)

What portions of the GI tract are affected by UC?

UC affects the rectum and may extend and involve the proximal colon

What portions of the GI tract are affected by Crohn's disease?

Any portion of the entire GI tract from mouth to anus (80% involve the distal ileum)

Do skip lesions characterize UC or Crohn's?

Crohn's

What are the risk factors for IBD?

Caucasian or Jewish ethnicity; Age 15–30 and 50–70 (bimodal age distribution); Female gender (for Crohn's disease) and male gender (for UC); Family history of IBD; Cigarette smoking (for Crohn's disease)

What genetic association does UC have?

UC has been associated with HLA DR2.

What are the typical symptoms of UC?

Bloody diarrhea with mucus passage and abdominal pain, possibly with tenesmus, fever, and weight loss

What are the typical symptoms of Crohn's disease?

Typically with a prolonged history of diarrhea; Crampy abdominal pain; Fatigue; Weight loss, with or without gross bleeding

In regards to toxic megacolon:

   What is it?

Complication of severe IBD (especially UC) or infectious colitis (especially *C. difficile*) when inflammation results in impaired colonic motility, colonic dilation, and decreased frequency of bowel movements

What class of medications may precipitate it?

Antidiarrheals

How does the patient present?

High fever; Leukocytosis; Abdominal tenderness; Rebound tenderness; Dilated segment of colon on abdominal XR

How is it treated?

Bowel rest; Nasogastric tube; IV fluids; Antibiotics to cover GI flora; Steroids if the cause is IBD

When is surgery required?

Perforation

What are the gastrointestinal complications of Crohn's disease?

Bowel perforation; Fibrotic strictures with resulting bowel obstruction; Abscess formation; Fistula formation; Anal fissures; Perirectal abscesses; Aphthous ulcers; Dysphagia

What are the extraintestinal complications of IBD?

Uveitis; Episcleritis; Erythema nodosum; Pyoderma gangrenosum; Peripheral arthritis; Ankylosing spondylitis; Sclerosing cholangitis; Venous thromboembolism

What endoscopic findings are consistent with a diagnosis of UC?

Continuous involvement of the colon, varying in severity from erythematous mucosa with petechiae and friability to macroulcerations and profuse bleeding

What biopsy findings are characteristic of UC?

Crypt abscesses and chronic changes such as atrophied glands and lost mucin in goblet cells

What endoscopic findings are consistent with a diagnosis of Crohn's disease?

Skip lesions, with focal ulcerations adjacent to normal mucosa, and a "cobblestone" appearance of polypoid mucosal changes

What biopsy findings are characteristic of Crohn's disease?

Focal ulcerations with both acute and chronic inflammation, and noncaseating granulomas in about 30% of patients

What features distinguish colon-involving Crohn's disease from ulcerative colitis?

Rectal sparing; Co-involvement of the small bowel; Lack of gross bleeding; Perianal involvement; Fistula formation; Granuloma presence; Focal lesions

What autoantibodies have been associated with IBD?	Perinuclear antineutrophil cytoplasmic antibody (P-ANCA) (in UC) and anti-saccharomyces cerevisiae antibody (ASCA) (in Crohn's disease), although accuracy and predictive value of these tests are unestablished
What medication is considered first-line therapy in IBD?	5-aminosalicylate (5-ASA) containing compounds
For what cases of IBD is sulfasalazine effective?	Since sulfasalazine is metabolized to 5-ASA and a sulfapyridine moiety in the colon, it is used for UC or Crohn's disease limited to the colon
What preparation of 5-ASA can be used for Crohn's disease involving the small bowel?	Mesalamine
When should glucocorticoids be used to treat IBD?	To induce remission in flare-ups of moderate to severe disease or mild disease that is unresponsive to 5-ASA or to treat extraintestinal manifestations. They are not used for maintenance therapy.
When should immunomodulating therapies be considered in treating IBD?	Immunomodulating agents such as 6-mercaptopurine, azathioprine, methotrexate, cyclosporine, and infliximab should be considered for refractory cases of IBD
When should surgery be considered for IBD?	Complications such as life-threatening bleeding, fistulas, obstruction, perforation, abscesses, and in medically refractory disease or neoplastic transformation
Is there an association between IBD and increased risk of colorectal cancer (CRC)?	Yes (related to extent and duration of the disease)
Is the risk higher with UC or Crohn's?	UC

COLORECTAL CANCER

In the United States, what is the third leading cause of cancer and cancer death in men and women?	CRC
What genetic disorders predispose a person to CRC?	FAP and HNPCC, along with variants such as Gardner's syndrome and Lynch syndrome

What is familial adenomatous polyposis (FAP)?

A familial colon cancer syndrome in which a germline mutation in the Adenomatous Polyposis Coli (APC) gene results in numerous colonic adenomas appearing during childhood

What percent of patients with FAP develop colon cancer?

90% by age 45

What is HNPCC (hereditary nonpolyposis colorectal cancer)?

A familial colon cancer syndrome associated with defects in DNA mismatch repair

What are other risk factors for CRC?

Age >40–50 years; Personal history of CRC; Personal history of polyps; First-degree relative diagnosed with CRC; IBD; Cigarette smoking

True or false: In most cases of CRC, there is a positive family history of the disease.

False

What is the most common presenting symptom of CRC?

Abdominal pain

What other symptoms may help localize the lesion to the:

Right side

Iron-deficiency anemia; Weight loss; Anorexia

Left side

Decreased stool caliber; Constipation; Obstipation; Diarrhea

Rectum

Bright red blood per rectum and/or tenesmus

Approximately what percent of patients are asymptomatic at the time of diagnosis?

33%

What is the diagnostic test of choice for patients with symptoms suggestive of CRC?

Colonoscopy

What if the colonoscope cannot reach the tumor site?

Double-contrast barium enema

What is the differential diagnosis of CRC?

Other malignancies (lymphoma, carcinoid, Kaposi's sarcoma, or metastases); Hemorrhoids; IBD; Diverticulitis; Infection

What are the most common sites of metastases of CRC?

Regional lymph nodes; Liver; Lungs; Peritoneum

What does the metastatic workup of CRC involve?

CXR; LFTs; Abdominal CT

Should carcinoembryonic antigen (CEA) be used as a screening test for CRC?	No
When do you use CEA?	In patients newly diagnosed with CRC, for both prognosis and evaluation
What is the most important prognostic factor in CRC?	Depth of bowel wall invasion
What is the only curative modality for localized CRC?	Surgical resection
Describe the adjuvant treatments for CRC.	Chemotherapy, when there are positive nodes; radiation in treatment in rectal cancer
For average-risk individuals, at what age should CRC screening begin?	50 years
What are the different options for CRC screening?	Fecal occult blood test (FOBT) every year; Flexible sigmoidoscopy alone every five years; Flexible sigmoidoscopy every five years with FOBT yearly; Double-contrast barium enema every five years; Colonoscopy every ten years
Which of the above has the greatest sensitivity and specificity?	Colonoscopy
What are some disadvantages to colonoscopy?	Risk of bleeding/perforation; Patient has to do bowel prep; Costly; Sedation leads to longer recovery time (and adds indirect costs for transportation, absenteeism)
What are some advantages to colonoscopy versus other types of screening?	Ability to localize lesions throughout the entire colon, biopsy mass lesions, and remove polyps
Describe CRC screening in the following patient populations.	
Patients with family history of first-degree relative with CRC	Colonoscopy every ten years starting at age 40 or ten years prior to the age at diagnosis of the youngest family member with CRC. Whichever comes first
Patients with inflammatory bowel disease	Colonoscopy every 1–2 years starting 8–10 years after diagnosis, or 15 years after diagnosis if disease is limited to the left colon

CHAPTER 5

Pulmonology

ASTHMA

What triad is associated with asthma?	1. Asthma 2. Eczema 3. Rhinitis
What is the pulmonary function test (PFT) pattern of asthma, obstructive or restrictive?	Obstructive
What does the abbreviation "FEV1" mean?	Forced expiratory volume in the first one second of expiration
What does the abbreviation "FVC" mean?	Forced vital capacity of the lungs
Describe the FEV1/FVC ratio typical of asthma.	Decreased FEV1/FVC (<80%), which improves with bronchodilator therapy
What are the most common symptoms of asthma?	Wheezing; Shortness of breath (SOB); Cough
What medications are commonly used for immediate relief of asthma symptoms?	Inhaled short-acting beta-2 agonists
What medications are commonly used for the prophylactic treatment of asthma symptoms?	Inhaled corticosteroids; Leukotriene modifiers; Cromolyn; Long-acting beta-2 agonists
What are typical signs of asthma exacerbation?	Tachypnea; Tachycardia; Cyanosis; Use of accessory muscles to breath; Wheezing
What is the treatment for an acute exacerbation?	Oxygen to a saturation of greater than 92%; Inhaled albuterol every 20 minutes (more often if severe); Inhaled ipratropium; Corticosteroids; Subcutaneous epinephrine for very severe exacerbation
Why is an elevated PaCO$_2$ of particular concern during an asthma attack?	Typically, patients hyperventilate during an attack and thus have a low PaCO$_2$, so an elevated PaCO$_2$ may indicate patient fatigue and impending respiratory failure

What is commonly used to quantify improvement of asthmatic symptoms on prophylactic medications?

Home peak flow monitoring

What is an asthma trigger?

Something that causes an exacerbation of asthma symptoms after exposure

What are some common asthma triggers?

Dust mites; Seasonal allergens; Smoke; Chemicals (i.e., perfume); Aspirin; Cold air; Stress; Pet dander

Describe the typical chest x-ray (CXR) of an asymptomatic asthma patient.

Normal

What does PEFR stand for?

Peak expiratory flow rate

What is the PEFR used for?

A patient's self-monitoring of lung function and trends

What is Churg-Strauss syndrome?

Asthma plus eosinophilia and granulomatous vasculitis

CHRONIC OBSTRUCTIVE PULMONARY DISEASE

What is chronic obstructive pulmonary disease (COPD)?

A respiratory illness with airflow limitation that is not completely reversible

What are the common clinical manifestations of COPD?

Cough; Dyspnea; Sputum production

What are typical CXR findings in a patient with COPD?

Usually normal, but in *advanced* disease you may see flattened diaphragms, enlarged lung fields, increased AP diameter, or interstitial markings with bullae

What are the typical findings on ECG?

Usually normal, but you may see poor R-wave progression in leads V1–V6, right-sided heart strain, or low-voltage QRS due to increased chest diameter

What are the two typical types of COPD?

Chronic bronchitis and emphysema

What is chronic bronchitis?

A chronic expiratory airflow obstruction with productive cough for at least three months in a year for two years

Is the term "blue bloater" used to describe patients with chronic bronchitis or emphysema?

Chronic bronchitis

Is the term "pink puffer" used to describe patients with chronic bronchitis or emphysema?

Emphysema

What is the definition of emphysema?

Chronic expiratory airflow obstruction with enlargement of the airspaces and destruction of alveoli

What are the typical PFTs findings associated with COPD?

Obstructive pattern; With a decreased FEV1/FVC ratio; Increased residual volume

Are these findings fully reversible with bronchodilator therapy?

No

What is the strongest risk factor associated with centrilobular emphysema?

Smoking

In what percentage of smokers does COPD develop?

10–15%

What are the important secondary and tertiary prevention strategies for COPD?

Smoking cessation; Oxygen therapy; Rehabilitation; Vaccines (pneumovax, flu)

What genetic risk factor is associated with developing panacinar emphysema?

Alpha-1 antitrypsin deficiency

What two treatments are the only ones shown to improve mortality in a COPD patient?

1. Oxygen therapy
2. *Smoking cessation*

What is the benefit of corticosteroids in a COPD patient?

They decrease exacerbations and are useful in an acute setting

Do corticosteroids slow the FEV1 decline of COPD?

No

What kinds of bronchodilators are used in the treatment of COPD?

Anticholinergics (ipratropium); Beta-agonists (albuterol); Sometimes methylxanthine

What are indications for long-term home oxygen therapy in patients with COPD?

Arterial PO_2 <55 mm Hg or saturation of oxygen of less than 88% by pulse oximetry, with or without hypercapnia; Or arterial PO_2 from 55 mm Hg to 59 mm Hg with evidence of cor pulmonale; Pulmonary hypertension; Congestive heart failure ([CHF] or an elevated hematocrit [>55%])

Can oxygen be prescribed to patients for exercise?

Yes. If their PO_2 drops to 55 mm Hg or less during exercise

In regards to an acute exacerbation of COPD, what is/are the:

Most common cause	Infection (particularly viruses [like influenza], *Streptococcus pneumoniae, and Moraxella catarrhalis*)
Secondary causes	Cardiac failure or arrhythmias; Chest trauma; Pneumothorax; Pulmonary embolism; Iatrogenic (inappropriate doses of beta-blockers, narcotics, etc.)
Symptoms of an exacerbation	Worsening dyspnea and increased sputum production
Workup	Arterial blood gases; CXR; ECG; Labs (CBC, BMP); Spiral CT if pulmonary embolism is suspected
Treatment	Oxygen—to maintain an O_2 saturation of at least 90–94%; Bronchodilator therapy; Corticosteroids; Antibiotics (especially if patient notes a change in sputum production or color)
Reason for monitoring PCO_2 while on O_2 therapy for an acute exacerbation	Oxygen can decrease the respiratory drive, causing the individual's PCO_2 to increase
Treatment available to deal with hypercapnia	BiPAP, then intubation if needed

What does "BiPAP" stand for?   Bi-level (variable) positive airway pressure

What does BiPAP do?   Mechanically delivers air through a mask at one pressure for inhaling (high) and at another for exhaling (low)

PNEUMONIA

What are some common symptoms of pneumonia?	Fever; Cough; Sputum production; Pleuritic chest pain; Dyspnea
What is the most common bacterial cause of pneumonia in adults?	*S. pneumoniae*
What patients are particularly prone to infection with *S. Pneumoniae*?	Those with splenectomy, sickle cell disease, lung disease, HIV, and/or renal failure
In an elderly patient, what other pathogens commonly cause pneumonia?	Influenza; Tuberculosis (TB); *Legionella*

In a young healthy adult, what other pathogens commonly cause pneumonia?	*Mycoplasma*; *Chlamydia*; Viruses
What is the most common cause of pneumonia in young children?	Respiratory viruses

What additional cause(s) of pneumonia should you keep in mind for a patient with a history of the following:

COPD	*H. influenzae*; *S. pneumoniae*; *M. catarrhallis*
Mechanical ventilation	*Pseudomonas aeruginosa*; *Acinetobacter*; *Methicillin-resistan Staphylococcus aureus (MRSA)*
Immune suppression	*Pneumocystis carinii*; Fungi; *Nocardia*; TB; Atypical mycobacteria
Seizures	Aspiration
Alcoholism	Aspiration; *Klebsiella*; *S. pneumoniae*; Gram-negative rods
Aspiration pneumonia	Gram-negative rods; Anaerobes; *S. aureus* (all present in the upper GI tract and upper airways)
Recent exposure to deer or rabbits	*Francisella tularensis* (Tularemia)
Residence or travel to the Southwest US	*Coccidioides immitis*
Prominent exposure to rodents	Hantavirus; Yersinia pestis
Exposure to cattle, goats, and/or sheep	Q fever; Brucellosis
Exposure to dog ticks	Ehrlichiosis
Who is at increased risk for developing pneumonia due to *S. aureus*?	Patients with viral pneumonia; Those infected by a hematogenous route (i.e., IV drug users or patient with infective endocarditis); Diabetics; Patients with liver disease
What are common sources for *Legionella*?	Air conditioners; Shower heads; Condensers
What populations are most susceptible to pneumonia from *Legionella*?	Elderly; Smokers; Immunocompromised
What symptoms are common in a patient with pneumonia secondary to *Legionella*?	Dry cough; Fever; Headache; Confusion; Weakness; GI disturbances (diarrhea)
What is the typical description for the sputum in *Klebsiella* infection?	Currant jelly sputum
Which patients are more prone to infection with *Pseudomonas*?	Patients with diabetes or cystic fibrosis

What kind(s) of pneumonia would you most suspect with the following CXR findings?

Lobar consolidation	Typical pneumonia
Diffuse, reticulonodular densities (the CXR looks "worse" than the patient)	Atypical pneumonia (i.e., due to *Mycoplasma*); and *Pneumosystis carinii pneumonia (PCP)*
Interstitial infiltrates	Virus
Prominence of the hilar region	TB; Virus; Fungus (also think of a possible malignancy)
Cavitations	*S. aureus*; Gram-negative rods; Anaerobes; TB
Bulging fissure sign	*Klebsiella*

What etiologies come to mind if your patient describes symptoms with a slow, insidious onset?

Fungi; TB; Anaerobic pathogens; Anatomical defects

Acute onset?

S. Pneumoniae; Mycoplasma; Viruses

A sputum sample is considered adequate when there are how many epithelial cells and polymorphonuclear (PMN) cells per high-powered field?

Less than 10 epithelial cells and more than 25 PMN cells

Should immunocompetent patients receive an influenza vaccine after they recover from a bout of pneumonia?

Yes

Why is hospital-acquired pneumonia usually more severe than community acquired pneumonia?

Patient debilitated due to original reason for admission and pneumonia is more likely to be an antibody-resistant variety

What causes chemical pneumonitis?

Aspiration of sterile gastric contents

What are the typical signs and symptoms of chemical pneumonitis?

Abrupt onset of dyspnea; Infiltrates on CXR involving dependent areas of lung; Low-grade fever

LUNG CANCER

What is the leading cause of cancer deaths in both men and women?

Lung cancer

What is the most prominent risk factor for developing lung cancer?

Smoking, including exposure to second-hand smoking

What lung cancer is typically located centrally?

Small cell and squamous cell

What type of lung cancer is considered sensitive to chemotherapy?	Small cell
What type of lung cancer is treated with surgery?	Squamous cell
Which lung cancer is not linked to smoking and is more common in women?	Bronchoalveolar adenocarcinoma
What is the most common symptom of lung cancer?	Chronic cough
What are other signs and symptoms of lung cancer?	Hemoptysis; Stridor; Dyspnea; Hoarseness; Dysphagia; Associated paraneoplastic syndromes
What is superior vena cava (SVC) syndrome?	A tumor obstructs venous blood flow in the SVC causing facial swelling, headaches, and dyspnea
What typically worsens the symptoms of a patient with SVC?	Lying down or sleeping
What are the three signs typical of Horner's syndrome?	1. Ptosis 2. Miosis 3. Anhidrosis
With which type of lung cancer do you more often see hypercalcemia?	Squamous cell lung cancer due to its association with parathyroid hormone-related protein (PTHrp)
With which type of lung cancer do you more often have problems with hyponatremia?	Small cell lung cancer due to association with syndrome of inappropriate antidiuretic hormone (SIADH)
What is cause of Eaton-Lambert Syndrome?	Antibodies attack presynaptic nerve terminals, thereby decreasing acetylcholine release
What are typical early signs of Eaton-Lambert syndrome?	Weakness of the hip girdle muscles with associated difficulty getting out of and into chairs
Do the symptoms of Eaton-Lambert typically worsen or improve as the day goes by?	Improve
How is lung cancer diagnosed?	Through imaging with CXR and CT, but biopsy gives the definitive diagnosis
What cancer is associated with asbestos exposure?	Mesothelioma

CHAPTER 6

Infectious Disease

HUMAN IMMUNODEFICIENCY VIRUS

What is the mechanism of HIV transmission?	Contact with infected blood and body fluids, or vertical transmission from mother to fetus
What screening test is used for HIV?	Enzyme-linked immunosorbent assay (ELISA)
What diseases can give a false positive HIV ELISA result?	Syphilis, Lyme disease, and systemic lupus erythematosus (SLE)
What confirmatory test is used for HIV?	Western blot
As per the US Preventive Services Task Force (USPSTF), who should get an HIV test (Grade A recommendation)?	Patients with increased risk for HIV infection; Patients receiving health care in a high-risk setting and/or where the prevalence of HIV is >1%; All pregnant women
What groups of patients are at increased risk for HIV infection (as well as their partners)?	Men who have sex with men; Persons who have unprotected sex with multiple partners, an HIV-infected partner, or a bisexual partner; Persons who exchange money or drugs for sex; Persons being treated for STDs; IV drug users; Persons who received a blood transfusion between 1978 and 1985
As per the Centers for Disease Control and Prevention (CDC), who should get an HIV test?	Regardless of risk factors all patients 13–64 years old (unless prevalence of undiagnosed HIV infection in patient population has been documented to be <0.1%); All pregnant women; All patients initiating treatment for TB; All patients seeking treatment for STDs

The CDC recommends "opt-out screening" for HIV. What does this mean?

All should be screened after being notified that they will be screened unless they decline

Is specially written consent needed for an HIV test?

In most states, yes (review your local laws). But recent CDC recommendations endorse allowing general consent for medical treatment to cover HIV testing

When should a pregnant woman get an HIV test during her pregnancy?

As soon as possible in the pregnancy

Under what circumstances should pregnant women get an additional HIV test during the third trimester?

Lives in an area with elevated incidence of HIV/AIDS (22 states in 2006); Has high risk for acquiring HIV; If there are symptoms consistent with acute HIV infection

Why is HIV-1 RNA viral load by polymerase chain reaction (PCR) a useful test in the following circumstances?

    Early HIV infection

ELISA and Western blot can be negative because antibodies have not been formed, but viral load is high

    HIV in neonates

Cannot use serologic tests since mother's antibodies are passed through placenta and would result in false positive tests

How does one monitor disease progression in HIV?

CD4 count; Viral load

What determines whether a patient has AIDS?

HIV + plus either CD4 count <200; Opportunistic infection; B-cell malignancy; Kaposi's sarcoma

What is the most common opportunistic infection in HIV patients?

Pneumocystis pneumonia (PCP)

What is the best predictor of an HIV patient's susceptibility to infection?

CD4 count

What infections is a patient susceptible to when the CD4 count is:

    <500?

Candida; TB; Herpes simplex virus (HSV); Varicella-zoster virus (VZV)

    <200?

PCP; *Toxoplasma; Cryptococcus; Histoplasma; Coccidioides; Bartonella*

    <50–100?

Mycobacterium avium complex (MAC); Cytomegalovirus (CMV);

Bacillary angiomatosis (disseminated *Bartonella*); CNS lymphoma; Progressive multifocal leukoencephalopathy (PML)

What is the most common cause of pneumonia in an HIV patient?

Streptococcus pneumoniae (same as in the immunocompetent population)

What is the differential diagnosis of pulmonary infection in an HIV patient?

See Table 6.1

What are the associated clinical features, diagnostic methods, and treatment of each condition?

Table 6.1 Pulmonary Infection in HIV

Condition	Clinical features	Diagnosis	Treatment
Community acquired pneumonia (usually Streptococcus pneumomia)	Lobar pneumonia; Rust-colored sputum; Often acute onset; patient has shaking chills	Gram stain of sputum; Blood culture	Quinolone or third-generation cephalosporin; Macrolides
Pneumocystis pneumonia	Bilateral patchy infiltrates on chest x-ray; Hypoxic with exercise	Detection of *Pneumocystis jiroveci* by silver stain or immuno-fluorescence	TMP[+]/SMX +/− steroids (esp-ecially if hypoxic)
Tuberculosis	Fever; Night sweats; Cough; Hemoptysis; CXR with cavi-tary upper lobe infiltrates	PPD (to diagnose previous infect-ion); Sputum AFB stain/culture	4-drug regimen: INH[‡] (and pyridoxine); PZA[§]; Rifam-pin; etham-butol
Fungal pneumonia	Fever; Cough; May have systemic features of fungal illness (e.g., skin involvement)	*Histoplasma*: Urine histo antigen; Serology; High (LDH*) *Cryptococcus*: Serum crypto antigen; Sero-logy *Coccidioides*: Serology	Treat severe infection with amphotericin B *Histoplasma*: itraconazole ; *Cryptococcus*: fluconazole ; *Coccidioides*: fluconazole

*LDH: lactate dehydrogenase
**SMX : sulfamethoxazole
[+]TMP: trimethoprim 5` monophosphate
[‡]INH: isoniazid
[§]PZA: pyrazinamide
‖ AFB: acid fast bacilli

What is the differential diagnosis of neurologic deficits in an HIV patient?	Cryptococcal meningitis; Toxoplasmosis; Central nervous system lymphoma; Neurosyphilis; PML
What is the differential diagnosis of ring-enhancing lesions on CT in an HIV + patient?	Toxoplasmosis; CNS lymphoma
What is the differential diagnosis of chronic diarrhea in an HIV patient?	Protozoal infection; MAC; CMV colitis; HIV colitis; Highly active antiretrovial therapy (HAART)-related
What is the differential diagnosis of odynophagia (painful swallowing) in an HIV patient?	*Candida*; CMV; HSV; HIV-related
What is the treatment of an HIV patient with odynophagia?	Treat empirically for esophageal candidiasis with fluconazole for ten days.
Which malignancies are more common in HIV patients?	B-cell malignancies such as lymphoma (Hodgkin's, non-Hodgkin's, primary CNS); Kaposi's sarcoma
Name the four classes of medication used in HAART?	1. Protease inhibitors (PIs) 2. Nucleoside reverse-transcriptase inhibitors (NRTIs) 3. Non-nucleoside reverse transcriptase inhibitors (NNRTIs) 4. Fusion inhibitors (FIs)

What are the most common side effects of:

PIs (ritonavir)	GI symptoms; Insulin resistance; Hyperlipidemia
NRTIs (AZT, ddI, 3TC)	Mitochondrial toxicity → Neuropathy; Myopathy; Pancreatitis; Hepatic steatosis; Lactic acidosis
NNRTIs (nevirapine, efavirenz)	Rash (Stevens-Johnson Syndrome in severe cases); Liver toxicity (note: resistance to one NNRTI confers resistance to entire class)
FIs (enfurvitide)	Injection site reaction

Name the idiosyncratic side effects of:

AZT	Macrocytic anemia
Abacavir	Hypersensitivity (rash → if reintroduced, may be fatal)
Efavirenz	CNS toxicity
Indinavir	Kidney stones

When is the appropriate time to initiate HAART?	The patient has AIDS; Symptomatic HIV infection; Asymptomatic infection with high viral load (>20,000) and/or low CD4 count (<350); And when the patient is ready to take on the responsibility
What is meant by the term "immune reconstitution syndrome"?	Paradoxical worsening of clinical status after initiating HAART due to recovery of immune system
What medications are given to HIV patients as prophylaxis for opportunistic infections, based on a CD4 count of:	
<200?	TMP / SMX DS daily (prophylaxis vs. PCP)
<150?	Itraconazole 200 mg daily (if in endemic area for histoplasmosis)
<100?	TMP / SMX DS daily (prophylaxis vs. toxoplasmosis)
<50?	Azithromycin 1250 mg every week (prophylaxis vs. MAC)
Which vaccinations should be provided to all HIV patients?	Hepatitis A; Hepatitis B; Pneumococcus; Influenza (except nasal flu vaccine); Tetanus
Which vaccinations should be avoided in HIV patients?	Vaccines which contain live virus: Measles, mumps, and rubella (MMR) (unless the patient is asymptomatic and with CD >200); Varicella; Nasal flu vaccine

TUBERCULOSIS

What does *Mycobacterium tuberculosis* (TB) look like under the microscope?	It is an acid-fast bacillus ("red snapper")
What are the risk factors for infection with TB?	HIV+; Known exposure to infected person; Incarceration; Homelessness; Nursing home residence; Immigration from endemic area
Describe the pathogenesis of primary TB.	Exposure to droplet nuclei; Organisms replicate in lungs in host macrophages; Travel hematogenously to seed organs. Primary disease if host defense cannot contain the infection

Primary disease is characterized by what radiologic findings?

Infection in mid-lung fields and Ghon complex

If a patient whose host defenses initially contained the TB infection becomes immunocompromised in the future, what are they at risk for?

Secondary (reactivation) TB

What findings are characteristic of secondary TB?

Infection of the lung apex or extrapulmonary site (meninges, pleura, vertebrae, lymph nodes)

Extrapulmonary TB in the vertebral bodies is known as what disease?

Pott's disease

Extrapulmonary TB in the cervical lymph nodes is known as what disease?

Scrofula

What is miliary TB?

Disseminated infection, seen in immunocompromised hosts

What are the typical symptoms of pulmonary tuberculosis?

Long-standing; Productive cough; Hemoptysis; Systemic symptoms such as fever, chills, night sweats, and weight loss

What is a PPD?

PPD is a purified protein derivative from TB that is injected intradermally to test for TB (delayed-type hypersensitivity reaction)

What does a "positive PPD" signify?

The patient has been previously infected with TB

Does a "negative PPD" guarantee that your patient was never infected with TB?

No. Some immunocompromised hosts will be anergic and cannot mount a delayed-type hypersensitivity reaction (may place a *Candida* control to avoid this predicament)

How is a PPD read?

Measure area of *induration* around the injection site 48–72 hours after placement

For a high-risk patient (HIV, abnormal CXR, contact with infected person), what size induration meets the criteria for a positive PPD result?

>5 mm

If they are intermediate risk (imprisoned, homeless, low socio-economic status, nursing home, health care worker, immigrant, BCG)?

Greater than 10 mm

If they have no risk factors?

Greater than 15 mm

What is BCG?	A relatively ineffective TB vaccine given in countries where TB is endemic. Can be cause of false positive PPDs
How do you diagnose active pulmonary TB infection?	Sputum AFB smear (need three negative smears to rule out TB); Sputum culture (takes weeks to grow); PCR (insensitive); CXR with apical cavitary lung lesions
If the PPD is positive, but the CXR is negative and there is no other evidence of active infection, what is this called?	Latent TB
How do you treat this?	INH alone for nine months
If the PPD is positive, and the CXR is positive, what is this called?	Active TB
What drugs are used to treat active TB?	RIPPE: **R**ifampin; **I**NH; **P**yridoxine (vitamin B_6) to prevent peripheral neuropathy; **P**ZA; **E**thambutol (or streptomycin if cannot tolerate)
What is the duration of treatment of active TB?	Treat with all drugs for two months, then just INH/PZA for four months (total of six months of treatment)
What are the side effects of the drugs used in the 4-drug TB regimen?	See Table 6.2

Table 6.2   The Side Effects of TB Drug

Drug	Side effect/s	What we can do about it
INH	Hepatitis	Check liver function tests(LFT), stop drug if clinically significant hepatitis develops; abnormal LFTs are common with INH therapy. Recommend that pt not drink alcohol while taking med
	Peripheral neuropathy	Give pyridoxine (vitamin B_6)
PZA	Hepatitis	Check LFTs
Rifampin	Induces P450, enhancing metabolism of other drugs	Patients on oral contraceptives should use alternative birth control while on rifampin
	Interferes with Protease Inhibitors	In HIV patients on PIs, use rifabutin instead
	Turns body secretions red (urine, tears)	Warn your patients!
Ethambutol	Optic neuritis	Regularly test visual acuity/color discrimination

What should you do if your patient fails to respond to the 4-drug regimen, or if susceptibility testing of the cultured organisms demonstrates resistance?	Contact a physician with special training in infectious disease to determine appropriate treatment
If you suspect your patient has pulmonary TB, what steps should be taken?	Respiratory isolation; HIV test; Sputum acid fast bacilli (AFB); CXR; Sputum culture
What is DOT?	Directly observed therapy, whereby public health officials monitor patients in the community to ensure compliance
What is respiratory isolation?	Patient placed in negative pressure room; All persons in contact with patient should wear an N95 mask

SYPHILIS

What is the causative organism of syphilis?	*Treponema pallidum*
How does primary syphilis present?	Chancre (painless firm ulcer with raised edges—*syphiLIS is painLESS*) for 2–6 weeks
When does secondary syphilis present?	4–10 weeks after healing of the chancre
What are the symptoms of secondary syphilis?	Rash; Fever; Malaise; Arthralgia; Myalgia; Condyloma lata (genital warts)
Describe the rash characteristic of secondary syphilis.	Maculopapular rash including the palms, soles, and mucous membranes
How does tertiary syphilis present?	Systemic organ involvement: CNS effects (meningitis, tabes dorsalis, paresis); Cardiovascular effects (aortic aneurysms, aortitis, aortic regurgitation); Gummas (granulomatous lesion usually found in skin and bone)
What are the laboratory tests used to diagnose syphilis?	Rapid plasma reagin (RPR)/Venereal Disease Research Laboratory (VDRL-nontreponemal screening tests); Fluorescent treponemal antibody absorption (FTA-ABS)/ Treponema pallidum particle agglutination assay (TP-PA—treponemal confirmation tests); VDRL should be used on cerebrospinal fluid (CSF) for neurosyphilis

How are primary and secondary syphilis treated?	One dose benzathine penicillin G IM
How is latent syphilis treated?	One dose benzathine penicillin G IM weekly × 3 weeks; If neurosyphilis, give IV for 2 weeks
What allergic reaction can result during treatment of syphilis?	Jarisch-Herxheimer reaction (fever, chills, myalgias, tachycardia, tachypnea, hypotension)
Which STIs produce genital ulcers?	Syphilis; Chancroid (*Haemophilus ducreyi*); Herpes simplex virus (HSV); *Lymphogranuloma venereum* (*Chlamydia trachomatis* LGV serotype); Granuloma inguinale/donovanosis (*Calymmatobacterium granulomatis*)
How do you differentiate between a chancre and chancroid?	Chancres: Single; Sharply demarcated; firm; Nontender with nontender bilateral lymphadenopathy
	Chancroids: Multiple; Irregular; Soft; Very tender; With unilateral tender lymphadenopathy

HERPES

With which types of clinical disease are HSV-1 and HSV-2 typically associated?	HSV-1: Oral-facial lesions HSV-2: Genital lesions; Aseptic meningitis
How does a primary infection of HSV-2 typically present?	Papular eruption with itching and tingling which becomes painful and vesicular, possibly with severe inguinal adenopathy and influenza-like symptoms
What is the incubation period for HSV-2?	3–6 days
How long does an untreated primary HSV-2 infection typically last?	2–4 weeks
Where do the herpes viral particles reside during latency periods?	In the sensory nerve ganglia
How does a recurrent herpes infection present?	At the same site as primary infection, but with fewer lesions that are less tender and last only 2–5 days
Do patients infected with herpes shed virus only when lesions are present?	No. Subclinical shedding occurs in up to 60% of those infected, and there is a 2% of shedding at any given time

| How is herpes diagnosed? | Demonstration of HSV antigens or DNA (by polymerase chain reaction [PCR]) in scraping; Tzanck smear of tissue scrapings; Tissue culture of scrapings; Serum HSV-1 and HSV-2 antibodies |

How is genital herpes treated?

| First episode | Oral acyclovir; Valacyclovir; Famciclovir for 10–14 days |
| Symptomatic recurrent | Oral acyclovir; Valacyclovir; Famciclovir daily |

MOLLUSCUM CONTAGIOSUM

Describe the appearance of molluscum contagiosum.	Small (2–5mm) dome-shaped; Pearly white papules with central umbilication, however can be flesh-colored or yellow
Where do the warts of molluscum contagiosum usually appear?	Inguinal area; Inner thighs; Around the external genitalia; Rarely on extragenital sites
How are molluscum contagiosum warts transmitted?	By sexual or close contact
What organism causes molluscum contagiosum?	A large DNA virus of the Poxviridae family
How long do molluscum contagiosum lesions last?	Six months to many years
How is molluscum contagiosum diagnosed?	Clinical appearance
How is molluscum contagiosum treated?	It does not have to be, but for cosmetic reasons or minor symptoms, curette, liquid nitrogen cryosurgery, or electrodesiccation can be used

PARASITIC INFECTIONS

| Which parasites can be transmitted through sexual or close contact? | *Sarcoptes scabiei; Phthirus pubis* (causes "crabs," actually is a louse); Also Giardia via anal intercourse |
| What should people infected with scabies or crabs do with their clothing? | Launder all contaminated clothing or linen in hot water and bleach |

Where are the lesions of scabies usually found?

Lower abdomen; Buttocks; Inner thighs; Genitalia; Finger webs; Ventral wrist fold; Underneath breasts; Belt line

How do the lesions of scabies typically appear?

Papules; Vesicles; Pustules; Wheals with elongated burrows

What is the first-line treatment for scabies?

Permethrin cream (Elimite)

How do you diagnose pediculosis pubis (crabs)?

Identifying nits or adult lice on the pubic hair shafts

How do you treat pediculosis pubis?

Permethrin cream applied for ten minutes is best; Kwell shampoo lathered for four minutes can be used, except during pregnancy or lactation

CHAPTER 7

Endocrinology

HYPERTHYROIDISM

Describe the clinical manifestations of hyperthyroidism.

Dermatologic	Sweating; Hair thinning; Onycholysis (separation of nail from nail bed); Increased peripheral blood flow leading to warm skin
Cardiovascular	Tachycardia; Wide pulse pressure; Systolic hypertension; Atrial fibrillation (in 10–20% of patients with hyperthyroidism)
Respiratory	Increased oxygen consumption and respiratory muscle weakness lead to dyspnea
Gastrointestinal	Increased basal metabolic rate and increased gut motility lead to weight loss and diarrhea
Hematologic	Plasma volume increases more than red blood cells (RBC) mass leading to normocytic anemia
Genitourinary	Urinary frequency and nocturia; In females, anovulatory infertility, oligomenorrhea, and amenorrhea
Musculoskeletal	Proximal muscle weakness; Tremor (best seen in the outstretched hands or in the tongue); Increased bone resorption leading to osteoporosis
Psychiatric	Anxiety

What is the best single lab test to assess thyroid function?   Thyroid-stimulating hormone (TSH)

Interpret these lab findings.

Elevated free T4 and low TSH	Hyperthyroidism
Normal free T4 and low TSH	Subclinical hyperthyroidism
What test should you order if the free T4 is elevated but TSH is normal or elevated?	MRI to look for a TSH-producing pituitary adenoma

Differentiate the causes of hyperthyroidism based on thyroid size.

Diffusely enlarged goiter	Graves' disease; Toxic multinodular goiter (in countries with low iodine intake)
Palpable nodule	Thyroid adenoma
Normal	Subacute thyroiditis; Exogenous hyperthyroidism (factitious vs. iatrogenic); Ectopic hyperthyroidism (struma ovarii)

What is struma ovarii?	Functioning thyroid tissue in an ovarian neoplasm
What physical findings are unique to Graves' disease?	Ophthalmopathy; Infiltrative dermopathy
Describe the ophthalmopathy seen with Graves' disease?	Stare; Lid lag; Exophthalmos
What is lid lag?	When a person with Graves' disease looks down, the upper sclerae can be seen since the upper eyelid closes slowly
What causes the exophthalmos in Graves' disease?	Eye pushed outward secondary to inflammation of the extraocular muscles and orbital fat
Describe the infiltrative dermopathy seen with Graves' disease.	Pretibial myxedema with raised, hyperpigmented, violaceous, orange-peel textured papules
Describe the pathology behind Graves' disease.	An autoimmune disorder characterized by TSH receptor antibodies
Besides the physical examination, how can you diagnose the cause of hyperthyroidism?	Radioactive iodine uptake (RAIU) scan
What does high radioiodine uptake indicate?	*De novo* hormone synthesis
Is treatment with radioiodine ablation or thionamides appropriate?	Either will work to decrease hormone synthesis.

What does low radioiodine uptake indicate?

Destruction of thyroid tissue with release of preformed hormone or an extrathyroidal source

Is treatment with radioiodine ablation or thionamides inappropriate?

No

What are the causes of high radioiodine uptake?

Graves' disease; Toxic adenoma; Toxic multinodular goiter; TSH-producing pituitary adnenoma; Beta-human chorionic gonadotropin β-hCG-mediated hyperthyroidism

What are the causes of beta-hCG-mediated hyperthyroidism?

Hydatidiform mole; Choriocarcinoma; Testicular germ cell cancer

Why does high beta-hCG cause hyperthyroidism?

β-hCG has some TSH-like activity due to their shared alpha subunit.

What are the causes of low radioiodine uptake?

Thyroiditis; Exogenous thyroid hormone; Ectopic thyroid

What is thyroiditis?

Transient hyperthyroidism secondary to the release of preformed hormones

What are some causes of thyroiditis?

Viral; Postpartum; Chemical (e.g. amiodarone induced); Post-radiation

How do you differentiate between the causes of subacute thyroiditis?

Subacute granulomatous thyroiditis is painful and viral, while subacute lymphocytic thyroiditis is painless and often postpartum

How do you treat the beta-adrenergic symptoms (such as tachycardia and tremor) of Graves' disease?

Propranolol

What are the main treatments of hyperthyroidism?

Thionamides (methimazole and prophylthiouracil); Radioactive iodine ablation (ablation within 6–18 weeks); Thyroidectomy

What supplementation will a patient need after undergoing ablation or surgery?

Levothyroxine

Which thionamide should be used during pregnancy?

Propylthiouracil

Why?

It crosses the placenta less during pregnancy

What characteristics would make you more concerned that a thyroid nodule was malignant?

History of neck irradiation; "Cold" nodule; Male sex; Firm and fixed solitary nodule

What is a "cold" nodule?	On radioiodine uptake (RAIU), the absence of uptake in one nodular region
What test should you order to evaluate a "cold" nodule?	Fine needle aspiration (FNA) of the nodule
How do you treat subacute thyroiditis?	Beta-blockers for hyperthyroidism or levothyroxine for hypothyroidism; Anti-inflammatory medications (aspirin, nonsteroid anti-inflammatory drugs [NSAIDs], or steroids)

HYPOTHYROIDISM

Describe the clinical manifestations of hypothyroidism.

Dermatologic	Decreased blood flow leads to cool, pale skin, coarse hair and brittle nails. Accumulation of glycosaminoglycans in interstitial spaces leads to nonpitting edema (i.e., myxedema)
Cardiovascular	Decreased heart rate and contractility lead to decreased cardiac output, which leads to dyspnea on exertion.
Gastrointestinal	Decreased motility leads to constipation and the combination of decreased basal metabolic rate and increasing edema leads to weight gain.
Hematologic	Decreased RBC mass leads to a normocytic anemia.
Reproductive	Both amenorrhea and menorrhagia are possible; and decreased fertility
Neurologic	Carpal tunnel syndrome and delayed deep tendon reflexes (DTR)
Metabolic	Decreased free water clearance leads to hyponatremia; and increased cholesterol and triglycerides
What is cretinism?	Congenital hypothyroidism causing mental retardation and impaired growth

Interpret these lab findings.

| Low free T4 and high TSH | Overt hypothyroidism |
| Normal free T4 and high TSH | Subclinical hyperthyroidism |

Low free T4 and low TSH	Secondary hypothyroidism (rare)
What are some of the conditions that can cause secondary hypothyroidism?	Pituitary macroadenoma; Sheehan's syndrome (pituitary infarct secondary to postpartum hemorrhage)
What is the most common cause of hypothyroidism?	Hashimoto's thyroiditis (chronic autoimmune thyroiditis)
Which autoantibodies mediate destruction of thyroid tissue in Hashimoto's thyroiditis?	Antithyroglobulin and antithyroid peroxidase antibodies
What are risk factors for developing Hashimoto's thyroiditis?	Female sex; Family history of autoimmune disorders
What are the iatrogenic causes of hypothyroidism?	Thyroidectomy; External radiation therapy; Radioiodine therapy
What medications can cause hypothyroidism?	Lithium; Amiodarone; Interferon alpha; Interleukin 2
True or False? Iodine deficiency can cause hypothyroidism.	True. Less than 100 mcg of iodine consumption per day is a risk factor
True or False? Iodine excess can cause hypothyroidism.	True. Excess iodine can inhibit the organification of T4 and T3 (Wolff-Chaikoff effect)
How do you treat hypothyroidism?	Synthetic L-thyroxine (T4) supplement
How do you measure response to hypothyroidism therapy?	Check TSH every 4–6 weeks until euthyroid
How do you treat myxedema coma?	L-thyroxine IV

PARATHYROIDS

What is the most common cause of hypercalcemia as an outpatient?	Parathyroid adenoma or hyperplasia
What is the level of parathyroid hormone (PTH) in this setting?	Inappropriately high
What is the most common cause of hypercalcemia as an inpatient?	Cancer (that secretes PTH-related peptide or is invading the bone)
What is the level of PTH in this setting?	Low

DIABETES MELLITUS

What is the mechanism for Type I diabetes mellitus (DM)?	Insulin deficiency
What is the mechanism for Type II DM?	Insulin resistance

Table 7.1   Type I and II DM Differences

	DM I	DM II
Age	Young (<20 years) at onset	Older (>40 years)*
Body Habitus	Lean	Obese
Autoimmunity	Yes	No
Risk for ketosis	Yes	Rare

* With increasing incidence of childhood obesity, incidence of DM II is increasing in younger persons.

What are the main differences between type I and type II in terms of age, autoimmunity, body habitus, and risk for ketosis?	See Table 7.1
Which autoantibodies can be positive in type I DM?	Anti-islet cell; Antiglutamic acid dehydrogenase antibodies
What are the classic symptoms in DM?	Polyuria; Polydipsia; Unexplained weight loss (insulin is anabolic); Blurry vision
How do you diagnose diabetes?	Any one of the following criteria: See Table 7.2
What do you do after an abnormal test?	Confirm the diagnosis on a subsequent day by using one of the three criteria.
What is prediabetes?	Impaired fasting glucose and/or impaired glucose tolerance
What is the clinical implication of prediabetes?	Increased risk for future development of diabetes mellitus and macrovascular disease (50% increased risk for myocardial infarction or stroke)

Table 7.2   Diabetes Diagnostic Criteria

	Fasting blood glucose (FBG) (fasting = no caloric intake > 8 hours)	Oral glucose tolerance test (OGTT) (2 hours after 75 gram glucose load)	Random glucose
Abnormal	>125	≥200	>200 + classic symptoms
	100–125 = Impaired fasting glucose (IFG)	140–199 = Impaired glucose intolerance (IGT)	126–200 → perform follow-up FBG
Normal	<100	<140	≤125

What is the clinical management of a patient with prediabetes?	Address risk factors, measure blood pressure and serum lipids, and rescreen for diabetes annually
What behavior changes should you encourage in a patient with prediabetes?	Smoking cessation; Weight loss (5–10%); Diet changes; Exercise (30 min/d, 5 d/week)
Why is it important to identify patients with prediabetes?	Lifestyle modifications can delay and even prevent progression to diabetes
What are the three main microvascular complications of diabetes?	1. Retinopathy 2. Nephropathy 3. Neuropathy
What are the three main macrovascular complications of diabetes?	1. Atherosclerosis 2. Cerebrovascular disease 3. Peripheral vascular disease
How frequently should diabetics be seen by an ophthalmologist?	Annually
What is the incidence of retinopathy in type 2 diabetics at 20 years after diagnosis?	50–80%
What is usually the first sign of diabetic kidney damage?	Microalbuminuria (30–300 mg albumin in 24-hour urine)
What class of medications can help reduce the risk of diabetic nephropathy?	Angiotensin-converting enzyme (ACE)-inhibitors
What are the different types of diabetic neuropathies?	Peripheral; Autonomic; Mononeuropathy (e.g., cranial nerve palsies)
Describe the manifestations of diabetic peripheral neuropathy?	Symmetric, distal sensory loss; Parasthesias
How do you test for diabetic peripheral neuropathy?	Use the monofilament to test for sensation
How should diabetics care for their feet?	Inspect feet daily for skin cracks and signs of infection between the toes; Avoid walking barefoot; Ensure shoes fit appropriately
What should you look for when examining the feet of diabetics?	Skin breaks; Early ulcers; Decreased pedal pulses; Delayed capillary refill; Bony deformities
Describe the manifestations of autonomic neuropathy?	Gastroparesis; Orthostatic hypotension; Impotence; Neurogenic bladder
What interventions did the UK Prospective Diabetes Study compare?	4000 type 2 diabetics were assigned to either intensive therapy

	(sulfonylurea, metformin, and/or insulin) or diet alone
What did the study show?	Intensive therapy caused a 1% fall in HbA1c that was associated with a 35% reduction in microvascular endpoints, an 18% reduction in myocardial infarction, and a 17% reduction in all-cause mortality
How is HbA1c formed?	Glucose irreversibly attaches to hemoglobin at a rate dependent on blood glucose
What does HbA1c represent?	The mean blood glucose concentration over the 120-day life span of RBCs (but it correlates best with mean blood glucose concentrations over 56–84 days)
What will falsely elevate HbA1c?	Any process that decreases RBC turnover (vitamin B_{12}, folate, or iron deficiency)
What will falsely decrease HbA1c?	Any process that increases RBC turnover (hemolysis, etc.)
How frequently should HbA1c be checked?	Every 3–4 months until at goal, then every six months
What is the goal for HbA1c?	HbA1c <7%
What is the treatment for type I DM?	Insulin replacement
What are the treatments for type II DM?	Weight loss (exercise and calorie-restricted American Diabetes Association [ADA] diet); Oral hypoglycemic medications; Exogenous insulin
What are the four classes of oral hypoglycemic agents, their mechanism of action, and most common side effects?	See Table 7.3
Sulfonylureas and metformin can each decrease fasting glucose by what percentage?	20%
Sulfonylureas and metformin can each decrease HbA1c by what percentage?	1–2%
After three years of monotherapy, what percentage of patients will require the addition of a second medication for glycemic control?	50%

Table 7.3   The Side Effects of Hypoglycemic Medications

	Mechanism of action	Side effects	Comments
Sulfonylureas (Glimepiride, Glyburide, Glipizide)	Increases insulin secretion by the beta cells	Hypoglycemia	
Metformin	Decreases hepatic glucose production	Lactic acidosis especially in patients with renal insufficiency, diarrhea, and nausea	Can cause weight stabilization/ reduction
Thiazolidinediones (e.g., rosiglitazone, pioglitazone)	Increases insulin sensitivity in muscle and fat cells	Liver toxicity and fluid retention (caution in patients with CHF*)	Often used in combination with other medications
Alpha-glucosidase inhibitors (e.g., acarbose and miglitol)	Inhibits intestinal conversion of carbohydrates to monosaccharides	Diarrhea and flatulence	

* CHF: Congestive heart failure

What is the blood pressure goal for diabetics?	SBP <130 and DBP <80
Why is blood pressure control important in diabetics?	A 10 mm Hg reduction in systolic BP is associated with a 12% risk reduction in any diabetes-related complication.
Name the different types of insulin and their approximate peak effect.	See Table 7.4

Table 7.4   Insulin Duration

Fast Acting	
Lispro	~1 hour
Regular insulin	~3 hours
Intermediate Acting	
Neutral Protamine Hagedorn (NPH)	~8 hours
Long Acting	
Ultralente	~24 hours
Glargine (Lantus)	~24 hours (peakless)

What is the metabolic syndrome definition?

1. Any three of the following: Abdominal obesity (waist circumference in men >40 in, women >35 in)
2. Serum triglycerides ≥150 mg/dL
3. Serum high-density lipoprotein (HDL) cholesterol <40 mg/dL in men and <50 mg/dL in women
4. Blood pressure ≥130/85 mm Hg
5. Fasting plasma glucose (FPG) ≥100 mg/dL

What are the clinical implications of having the metabolic syndrome?

Increased risk of developing diabetes and cardiovascular disease

What is the body mass index (BMI) measurement?

Measurement of body fat based on height and weight; $((\text{weight in pounds})/(\text{height in inches})^2) \times 703$

Which BMI level represents being overweight?

Between 25 and 30

Which BMI level represents being obese?

≥30

What is gestational diabetes?

Impaired glucose tolerance in pregnant women because of increased anti-insulin hormones (estrogen and cortisol) and inadequate insulin production to meet the increased demands

How do you treat gestational diabetes?

Changes in diet and, if necessary, insulin

Is gestational diabetes a risk factor for developing diabetes in the future?

Yes

Which diseases of the exocrine pancreas can cause diabetes?

Cystic fibrosis; Hemochromatosis; Chronic pancreatitis

Which endocrinopathies can cause diabetes?

Any increase in hormones that inhibit insulin; Cushing's (cortisol), glucagonoma (glucagon), pheochromocytoma (epinephrine), and acromegaly (growth hormone)

What is diabetic ketoacidosis (DKA)?

A medical emergency where insulin deficiency leads to hyperglycemia, electrolyte disturbances, ketonemia, and metabolic acidosis

How does the insulin deficiency precipitate DKA?

In insulin deficiency, the liver breaks down lipids into ketone bodies resulting in a decrease in blood pH (serum ketones + acidosis)

What can precipitate DKA?	The four Is: Infection; Infarction (myocardial); Insulin deficiency; Idiopathic. Consider medication noncompliance, cerebrovascular accident (CVA), and physical stress
How do you categorize the acid-base abnormality in DKA?	Anion gap metabolic acidosis with compensatory respiratory alkalosis
What is Kussmaul's breathing?	Rapid, deep breathing to help increase CO_2 excretion and correct the underlying acidosis in DKA
A patient with DKA can have what odor to their breath?	Fruity; Acetone odor
What is the treatment of DKA?	Aggressive IV fluids; IV insulin; Replacement of electrolytes (potassium, phosphorus)
When can you transition the patient from IV insulin to subcutaneous insulin?	When the anion gap has resolved and the bicarbonate level approaches normal
What is hyperosmolar nonketotic (HONK) state?	Seen in type II diabetes with blood glucose generally >600, serum osmolality usually >350 mOsm/L, and no ketones
How do you treat HONK?	Aggressive IV fluids and insulin if needed

CHAPTER 8

Otolaryngology

COMMON COLD

What is the leading cause of work and school absenteeism?	Common cold
What causes most acute upper respiratory infections (URIs)?	Viruses (i.e., rhinovirus, coronavirus)
What is the primary mechanism of transmission?	Hand-to-hand contact
How long do colds last?	10–14 days, but can last up to a month (important to tell patients)
What are the symptoms of a cold?	Fatigue; Mild myalgias; Nasal congestion; Rhinorrhea; Sneezing; Coughing
What are the clinical signs of a cold?	Low-grade fever; Erythematous and swollen nasal mucosa; Nasal discharge
What does colored (brown, yellow, or green) versus clear nasal discharge indicate?	Inflammation (still most likely viral, not necessarily a secondary bacterial infection)
What are some conservative supportive measures in the treatment of colds?	Rest; High fluid intake; Saline drops; A humidifier (to loosen secretions)
What pharmacologic agents can be used for symptomatic relief of a cold?	Acetaminophen or ibuprofen for fever and headache; Pseudoephedrine for congestion and rhinorrhea; Dextromethorphan/guaifenesin for cough
Are antibiotics helpful in treating the common cold?	No
The widespread practice of prescribing antibiotics for the common cold has led to what problem?	Multidrug resistant respiratory pathogens and the general public's expectation of receiving antibiotics for a cold

What are the potential complications of a cold?	Sinusitis; Otitis media; Lower respiratory tract infection; Exacerbation of asthma/chronic obstructive pulmonary disease (COPD)

RHINOSINUSITIS

What is rhinosinusitis?	Inflammation of one or more of the paranasal sinuses
How does it develop?	Nasal passage edema (usually due to infection) causes obstruction of the sinus ostia
What other factors may contribute to the development of rhinosinusitis?	Allergies; Anatomic abnormalities (e.g., nasal polyps, septal deviation, adenoidal hypertrophy); Foreign bodies; Irritants (e.g., tobacco); Dental infections
What systemic diseases may predispose a patient to recurrent or persistent rhinosinusitis?	Cystic fibrosis; Kartagener's syndrome; Immunodeficiency syndromes
When does the incidence of rhinosinusitis peak?	Winter
What are the signs and symptoms of rhinosinusitis?	High fever; Purulent nasal discharge; Facial pain/pressure; Ability to smell is decreased/lost (hyposmia/anosmia); Maxillary toothache; Painful mastication; Halitosis; Periorbital edema; Nocturnal cough
What is the "double sickening" phenomenon?	Biphasic illness: patient begins to improve from a URI but then acquires a secondary bacterial acute rhinosinusitis
What findings may help distinguish between a bacterial and viral infection?	Bacterial: unilateral sinus pain; Maxillary tooth pain; Persistence of symptoms for greater than seven days; Double sickening
By definition, what is the duration of acute rhinosinusitis?	Greater than three days but less than four weeks
Subacute	4–12 weeks
Chronic	Greater than three months
What other conditions may mimic sinus pain?	Migraine headaches; Nasal polyps; Dental abscesses; Temporal arteritis

What are the usual bacterial causes of rhinosinusitis?	*Streptococcus pneumoniae; Haemophilus influenza; Moraxella catarrhalis*
What kind of pathogens are the usual cause of rhinosinusitis resulting from a spreading dental infection?	Microaerophilic or anaerobic bacteria
What is the initial treatment of acute sinusitis?	Symptomatic treatment (i.e., decongestants and steroid nasal sprays)
Under what circumstances should antibiotics be used to treat acute sinusitis?	Patients with unresolved symptoms (maxillary or facial pain, purulent nasal discharge) despite decongestants and analgesics for seven days
Under what circumstances would you not wait for seven days?	Patients with severe illness (fever, facial erythema) need hospitalization for IV antibiotics
What are the first-line antibiotics for outpatient treatment (assuming the patient has not been on antibiotics in the previous month)?	High-dose amoxicillin; Extended release amoxicillin-clavulanate; Cefdinir; Cefpodoxime; Cefprozil; Telithromycin for ten days
What antibiotics are available for patients with a penicillin allergy?	Telithromycin; Clarithromycin; Azithromycin; Trimethoprim-sulfamethoxazole doxycycline; Quinolones (avoid for patients under 18 years)
What antibiotics are available in the setting of resistance to first-line therapy (or for patients who have been on antibiotics in the previous month)?	Extended release amoxicillin-clavulanate for mild to moderate disease and quinolones for severe disease
Are antibiotics effective treatment for chronic sinusitis?	No (get an otolaryngology consultation)
Under what circumstances should surgery be considered in the treatment of sinusitis?	Patients with more than three attacks in one year; Chronic sinusitis; Unresponsiveness to antibiotics; Anatomic abnormalities amenable to surgery
What is functional endoscopic sinus surgery?	A procedure that removes blockage at the sinus ostia and improves drainage and ventilation in most patients
Are imaging studies helpful in the initial evaluation of sinusitis?	No (except in uncertain or recurrent cases)
Under what circumstances is a CT scan indicated?	To establish a diagnosis of chronic rhinosinusitis; Workup a

	pre-operative patient; Or obtain more information when medical management has failed
Complications of rhinosinusitis are uncommon, however occur more frequently in which patient populations?	Children and patients with immunodeficiency disorders
What are the potential complications of rhinosinusitis?	Mucocele or mucopyoceles; Preseptal or orbital cellulitis; Orbital or brain abscess; Cavernous or sagittal sinus thrombosis; Meningitis; Encephalitis; Subdural empyema; Osteomyelitis
When must a patient with rhinosinusitis be promptly evaluated for complications?	Patient exhibits ocular or central nervous system (CNS) signs and symptoms
In what sinus do mucoceles most frequently occur?	Frontal sinus
How does the patient present?	Displaced eye; Diplopia
What population is most prone to orbital complications?	Children with ethmoid rhinosinusitis
What are the signs of orbital cellulitis?	Swelling and inflammation of the eyelids and proptosis
What are the signs of an orbital abscess?	Unilateral ophthalmoplegia and impairment of vision and conjunctival swelling
What are the signs of cavernous sinus thrombosis?	Bilateral ophthalmoplegia; Conjunctival swelling; Retinal engorgement; Fever

ALLERGIC RHINITIS

What is the most common cause of chronic rhinitis?	Allergic rhinitis
What are some other causes of chronic rhinitis?	URI; Idiopathic rhinitis (i.e., vasomotor rhinitis, autonomic hyperresponsiveness); Atrophic rhinitis; Rhinitis medicamentosum from drug withdrawal (e.g., cocaine, OTC decongestant nasal sprays); Nasal foreign bodies
What are the common symptoms of allergic rhinitis?	Sneezing; Rhinorrhea; Nasal congestion; Nasal and conjunctival itching; Cough (secondary to post-nasal drip); Asthma exacerbation

What allergens typically cause seasonal allergies?	Pollens and mold spores
What allergens typically cause perennial allergies?	Dust mites; Mold spores; Cockroach feces; Pet dander
What is the primary "treatment" of allergic rhinitis?	Avoidance of allergens
What symptoms are antihistamines helpful in reducing?	Sneezing; Rhinorrhea; Nasal; Ocular pruritis
Are antihistamines effective in relieving nasal congestion?	Generally, no
What are some available second-generation antihistamines?	Loratadine; Desloratadine; Fexofenadine; Cetirizine
In what ways are these superior to first-generation antihistamines?	Less likely to cause side effects (drowsiness, fatigue, dry mouth, urinary retention) and some come in an antihistamine-decongestant combination
In what ways are they *not* superior?	Not more effective, yet are more expensive and often require a prescription
Are steroid nasal sprays effective in relieving nasal congestion?	Yes
What are some available steroid nasal sprays?	Beclomethasone; Flunisolide; Fluticasone; Triamcinolone acetonide; Budesonide
What other kinds of nasal sprays are available and are more effective for rhinorrhea than nasal congestion?	Mast cell stabilizing agents (e.g., cromolyn sodium) and anticholinergic agents (e.g., ipratropium bromide)
Which patients should undergo allergen skin testing?	Patients with moderate to severe symptoms or perennial allergies; Who have failed medical treatment; Who need guidance for appropriate avoidance measures or immunotherapy
What medications should be withheld before allergen skin testing?	Methylxanthines; Beta-blockers; Antihistamines
What does radioallergosorbent (RAST) testing measure?	Allergen-specific IgE levels
What is immunotherapy (aka desensitization)?	Patient receives weekly injections with gradually increasing doses of antigens and over time the IgE response diminishes

| What class of antihypertensives should be avoided during immunotherapy? | Beta-blockers |
| How long should immunotherapy be administered to avoid recurrence of symptoms? | 3–5 years |

ACUTE OTITIS MEDIA (AOM)

What is AOM?	Middle ear inflammation associated with an infection
How is it thought to develop?	Dysfunction and/or inflammation of the eustachian tube causes inadequate ventilation of the middle ear resulting in a negative pressure that pulls up fluid and infectious agents
Name the causes of eustachian tube dysfunction/inflammation.	URI; Allergies; Enlarged adenoids; Irritants (i.e., tobacco smoke); Genetic factors
What are the symptoms?	Earache; Decreased hearing; Fever; Nausea; Vomiting
Why are symptoms alone not enough to make a diagnosis and why?	There is no one symptom that is found reliably in all patients with AOM
What does visualization of the tympanic membrane (TM) reveal?	Bulging, red, dull or opaque TM; Displaced or absent light reflex; Loss of bony landmarks; Impaired TM mobility
Which of these is the most important in diagnosis?	TM mobility
Does an erythematous TM indicate AOM?	Not necessarily (since increased intravascular pressure can also cause the TM to redden, such as when a child is crying)
What is the peak age of onset of AOM?	Six months to seven years
What is the peak season of AOM?	Winter (because of increased URIs)
What are the most common bacterial causes of AOM?	*S. pneumonia; H. influenza; M. catarrhalis*
What is the treatment for AOM?	Analgesic and antibiotic
What is the first-line antibiotic?	High-dose amoxicillin (for children, this means 70–90 mg/kg/day vs. standard 40 mg/kg/day)

True or false: Most cases of AOM will resolve spontaneously within 10 days without antibiotics? — True. In many countries, antibiotics are not used to treat AOM

Almost every AOM is followed by otitis media with effusion (fluid in the middle ear). How long may it take for the effusion to clear? — Up to three months

By definition, what is recurrent otitis media? — Three or more episodes of acute AOM in a six-month period or four or more in 12 months

What are the treatment options? — Antibiotic prophylaxis or surgery (tympanostomy tubes)

What antibiotics can be used for prophylaxis? — Amoxicillin and sulfisoxazole

How do tympanostomy tubes help prevent recurrence? — Ventilate and equalize pressure in the middle ear

What are the complications of AOM? — Hearing loss; Mastoiditis; Cholesteatoma; CNS infections; Thrombosis

OTITIS EXTERNA

What is otitis externa (OE)? — Infection of the ear canal ("swimmer's ear")

What is the peak season of OE? — Summer

What are the signs and symptoms of OE? — Earache; Canal is red and edematous and has purulent drainage; Movement of tragus is very painful

What are the most common causes of OE? — Pseudomonas sp.; S. Aureus

What antibiotics may be used to treat OE? — Ofloxacin; Polymyxin B/neomycin/ hydrocortisone; Ciprofloxacin/ hydrocortisone ear drops; Oral dicloxacillin for acute disease

When should you avoid neomycin? — When the TM is ruptured

How can the patient help prevent recurrences of OE? — Drying canals with alcohol drops (1/3 white vinegar, 2/3 rubbing alcohol), then acidifying with 2% acetic acid solution or using antibiotic drops

What is malignant otitis externa? — Invasive cellulitis around the ear most often occurring in diabetics and immune compromised patients (HIV, chemotherapy)

What causes it?

Pseudomonas aeruginosa in >90%

How is it treated?

Ciprofloxacin (early disease); IV antibiotics; Surgical debridement (severe disease)

Why should you scan the patient's head (either CT or MRI)?

To rule out osteomyelitis

PHARYNGITIS

What is pharyngitis?

Inflammation of the pharynx; Hypopharynx; Uvula; Tonsils

What are some noninfectious causes of pharyngitis?

Trauma; Smoke inhalation; Pollutants; Allergies; Gastroesophageal reflux

What is the most common infectious cause of pharyngitis?

Respiratory viruses (e.g., adenovirus, rhinovirus)

What other viruses can cause pharyngitis?

Coxsackievirus; Herpesvirus; Epstein-Barr virus (EBV) (infectious mononucleosis)

Of coxsackievirus, herpesvirus, and EBV, which is characterized by the following?

Erythematous-based small vesicles or ulcers in the pharynx and on the palms and soles

Coxsackievirus (known as hand, foot, and mouth disease)

Shallow, erythematous-based small vesicles, and ulcers on the gingival, vermillion border, and/or pharynx

Herpesvirus

Exudative tonsillitis, pharyngitis (for more than 10–14 days), cervical lymphadenopathy, fever, fatigue, and hepatosplenomegaly

Infectious mononucleosis (IM)

What test can be used to diagnose IM?

Monospot test (detects heterophile antibodies)

What other tests should be performed in patients with IM?

Liver function test (LFT); Complete blood count (CBC) and platelets; Coombs' test

What are the complications of IM?

Hepatitis; Ruptured spleen; Low blood cell counts; CNS infections

What precaution should patients take to reduce the risk of splenic rupture?	Avoid contact sports and heavy lifting in the first 2–3 weeks of illness
What nonviral pathogens can cause pharyngitis?	Group A beta-hemolytic streptococcus (GABHS); *Chlamydia trachomatis; Mycoplasma; Corynebacterium diphtheriae, M. tuberculosis; Neisseria Gonorrhea; Candida*
What is the only cause of pharyngitis that requires antibiotic treatment?	GABHS ("strep throat")
In what season is GABHS most common?	Winter and early spring
At what age is it most common?	3–10 years
What are the signs and symptoms of strep throat?	Sore throat; Dysphagia; Exudative tonsillitis; Fever (>38°C); Tender cervical lymphadenopathy; *Lack* of URI symptoms (cough, rhinorrhea)
How long does a GABHS infection cause a sore throat?	Less than a week (longer than that probably means that it is something else)
Is exudative tonsillitis unique to GABHS?	No (also present in adenovirus, coxsackievirus, and EBV infections)
What is the test of choice for diagnosing strep throat?	Rapid streptococcal antigen test
What test should be done if the rapid strep test is negative but clinical suspicion remains high?	Throat culture on blood agar plate (BAP)
What is the treatment of choice for GABHS?	Oral penicillin V potassium for ten days or a one-time dose of penicillin G benzathine IM
If the patient has a penicillin allergy?	Macrolides (clarithromycin, azithromycin, etc.) or clindamycin
Why might antibiotic treatment be unsuccessful?	Non-compliance or missed diagnosis of IM
What are the complications of GABHS?	Rheumatic fever (and subsequent heart valve damage); Peritonsillar abscess; Acute poststreptococcal glomerulonephritis (APSGN)
What are some signs and symptoms of rheumatic fever?	Carditis; Erythema marginatum; Migratory Polyarthritis; Subcutaneous skin nodules; Chorea; Fever
What are the signs and symptoms of peritonsillar abscess?	Worsening sore throat; Fever; Odynophagia/dysphagia; Difficulty

	speaking; Large tonsils; Displaced palate; Deviated uvula
How is it treated?	Drainage (with 18-gauge needle or surgically) and antibiotics (clindamycin or second- or third-generation cephalosporin)
What are the signs and symptoms of APSGN?	Edema; Hypertension (HTN); Gross hematuria; Oliguria; But at least half of patients are asymptomatic
What is the prognosis?	95–98% of patients recover fully
What is the typical latent period between GABHS infection and APSGN?	7–21 days (average = 10)

CHAPTER 9

Dermatology

SUPERFICIAL FUNGAL INFECTIONS

What are the different types of cutaneous fungal infections?	Superficial, deep (subcutaneous), opportunistic, and systemic fungal infections with cutaneous manifestations
Which two groups of organisms comprise the majority of superficial fungal infections?	Dermatophytes and yeasts
How can superficial fungal infections be diagnosed in the office using microscopy?	Combine loose hair, scale, or subungual debris with 1–2 drops of 10–20% KOH on a slide. Gently heat the slide and examine under low power for hyphae (septate, branching, rod-shaped fungal elements). Chlorazol black E (a fungal stain) can assist with hyphae visualization
What is a dermatophyte?	A fungus capable of living on the keratin found in hair, skin, and nails
What three species of fungi are referred to as dermatophytes?	1. *Microsporum* 2. *Trichophyton* 3. *Epidermophyton*
What is a synonym for superficial dermatophyte infections?	"Tinea" infections
How are these infections classified?	According to their anatomic location: Tinea capitis (scalp); Tinea faciei (face); Tinea barbae (beard); Tinea corporis (trunk and extremities); Tinea cruris (groin); Tinea manum (hands); Tinea pedis (feet); Tinea unguium (nails)
How does tinea corporis classically present?	Well-demarcated scaling plaque with a red, elevated, advancing border and an area of central clearing

(ringworm); and may include
pustules and vesicles at the margins

**Which dermatophyte is the most common
cause of superficial fungal infections?**

Trichophyton rubrum

**What is the most common cause of tinea
capitis in the United States?**

Trichophyton tonsurans infections

**What are the four classic clinical presen-
tations of tinea capitis?**

1. Seborrheic (scaly dandruff)
2. Black-dot (patches of "black-dot
   alopecia" as hairs are broken at
   the scalp surface)
3. Kerion (a tender boggy mass with
   enlarged posterior cervical lymph
   nodes)
4. Favus (oval patches of alopecia
   with a golden crust)

**What is the preferred treatment for tinea
capitis?**

Oral griseofulvin for at least four
weeks

**Describe the three clinical patterns of
tinea pedis?**

1. Interdigital—scaling, erythema, and
   fissuring in web spaces between
   toes
2. Moccasin-type—scaling and hyper-
   keratosis on soles and lateral feet
3. Inflammatory or vesiculobullous—
   vesicles on the arc and lateral
   aspect of the feet

**What type of tinea infection is often
associated with a dermatophyte id
reaction?**

Tinea pedis can result in a
generalized immunologic reaction
producing a vesicular eruption at
distant sites (i.e., hand dermatitis)
that resolves with treatment of the
primary infection

**Excluding tinea capitis and tinea unguium,
what is an appropriate treatment approach
for most tinea infections?**

Topical therapy with fungicidal
allylamines (terbinafine or naftifine)

How is tinea unguium treated?

Griseofulvin (long-term therapy can
cause liver problems); Itraconazole;
Terbinafine

**What are the potential complications of
using combined steroid-antifungal agents?**

Skin atrophy; Steroid-induced acne;
Striae

**Name two tinea infections not caused by
dermatophytes and name their respective
organisms.**

1. Tinea versicolor—*Pityrosporum
   orbiculare* or *Malassezia furfur*
2. Tinea nigra—*Phaeoannellomyces
   werneckii*

How does tinea versicolor present?	Hypopigmented or hyperpigmented erythematous macules with fine scale predominantly on the trunk
What is seen with a KOH preparation of tinea versicolor?	A "spaghetti and meatball" pattern with short hyphae and yeast
Describe the clinical pa. ˉ for these presentations of cutaneous c. ˈdiasis?	
Candidal intertrigo	Well-demarcated confluent pustules on an erythematous base with satellite ˈıles at the periphery within skin folu.
Thrush	Adherent, ˏ ˉe cheese-like plaques on the oral muc.
Perleche	Angular cheilitis with ˏ ˈhema, fissuring at the corner of u. ˈouth
Paronychia	Infection of the proximal nail fo. ˈhat presents with tenderness, erythema, and hyperkeratosis
What is the preferred topical therapy for superficial candidal infections?	Nystatin
Name three cutaneous infections that should be considered when evaluating a groin rash.	1. Tinea cruris (scale) 2. Candidal intertrigo (satellite pustules) 3. Erythrasma (corynebacterium fluoresces coral-red on Wood's lamp examination)

URTICARIA

How do urticarial lesions (hives) typically present?	Pruritic, raised, erythematous plaques with or without central pallor that can enlarge and coalesce
What is the hallmark of urticarial lesions?	Lesions disappear within a few hours after onset without leaving any residual marks
Name four systemic diseases in which urticaria can be a presenting sign.	1. Urticarial vasculitis 2. Systemic lupus erythematosus 3. Autoimmune thyroid disease 4. Cryoglobulinemia
How is angioedema different from urticaria?	Angioedema is deeper in the dermis and subcutaneous tissues resulting in more extensive swelling and edema

What is the time-course of acute urticaria and chronic urticaria?

Acute urticaria resolves within several hours and lasts less than six weeks. Chronic urticaria is present on most days and lasts for more than six weeks

Name the two classes of antibiotics that are most frequently implicated in causing antibiotic-induced urticaria.

1. Beta-lactam
2. Sulfa-containing antibiotics

Generalized urticaria following an insect sting should raise concern for what type of potentially life-threatening reaction with a future sting?

Anaphylaxis

How should you manage these patients?

Inform the patient about this risk, and ensure that they have epinephrine with them at all times

Describe four types of physical urticarias.

1. Immediate pressure—presents as dermatographism, often at sites of constricting undergarments
2. Delayed pressure—often affects the hands and feet
3. Cold
4. Cholinergic—punctuate, pencil-eraser-sized wheals in response to exercise, sweating and/or hot showers

What are the characteristic features of urticarial vasculitis?

Painful rather than pruritic wheals that persist beyond 24 hours and leave a residual pigmentation

Does urticarial vasculitis tend to respond to corticosteroids?

No

Describe the main treatment of urticaria.

Remove the offending trigger

What is the treatment of urticaria if the offending trigger is unknown or if symptoms persist even after removing the inciting agent?

Antihistamine H1-receptor blockers; H2-receptor blockers as adjunctive therapy; Short-term course of systemic steroids for patients who fail antihistamine therapy

CONTACT DERMATITIS

Name the two types of contact dermatitis.

Irritant and allergic

What is the pathophysiology of irritant contact dermatitis?

A high concentration of an external agent causes a nonimmunologic inflammatory reaction in the skin

Is contact dermatitis confined to the site of exposure?	Yes
What type of hypersensitivity reaction is allergic contact dermatitis?	Type IV; T-cell mediated
Is allergic contact dermatitis confined to the site of exposure?	No. It can be generalized
Should an exposure to an external agent resulting in an urticarial eruption be considered an allergic contact dermatitis?	No. Since it involves a specific IgE-mast cell interaction resulting in the release of vasoactive compounds that produce wheals, angioedema, and anaphylaxis
Is a latex-glove allergy an allergic contact dermatitis or an allergic contact urticaria?	Allergic contact urticaria
How is allergic contact urticaria diagnosed?	Prick test
Describe this test.	A small amount of allergen is injected subcutaneously and is positive if a wheal develops within 15–20 minutes
What is the key to diagnosing contact dermatitis?	A thorough history in combination with the location and distribution of the lesions
What is the most common allergen in allergic contact dermatitis in the United States?	Poison ivy
Which topical antibiotic is a common cause of contact dermatitis?	Neomycin-containing topical antibiotics

ATOPIC DERMATITIS

What is the atopic triad?	1. Asthma 2. Allergic rhinitis 3. Atopic dermatitis (eczema)
What is the clinical significance of the triad?	The presence of one of these disorders is believed to result in a genetic predisposition to other atopic disorders either in the same patient or in the patient's family members
What is meant by the term "eczematous?"	Presence of erythema, scaling, crusting, and oozing of serous fluid
True or false: In atopic dermatitis, a rash first appears and subsequently becomes itchy.	False. Atopic dermatitis is the itch that rashes, not the rash that itches

Describe the characteristic presentation of eczema in the following age groups.

Infants	Pruritic erythematous papules and vesicles that ooze and crust on the cheeks, forehead, and scalp (spares the diaper area)
Children	Lichenified scaly patches and plaques that ooze and crust on the wrists, ankles, buttocks/posterior thighs, and the antecubital and popliteal fossae
Adolescents	Scaling plaques on the face, neck, upper arms, back, and flexural creases
Adults	Scaling plaques on the hands, face, and neck

Describe some additional physical findings associated with atopic dermatitis.	Xerosis (dry skin); Infraorbital skin folds (Dennie-Morgan lines); Bluish discoloration of the periorbital skin; Hyperlinear palm and sole creases; Keratosis pilaris (follicular accentuation on the posterolateral arms and anterior thighs)
Name some common food allergens that have been associated with atopy.	Milk; Egg whites; Wheat; Soy; Peanuts
Can atopic dermatitis be cured?	No. They can only be managed
Describe a rational treatment approach for atopic dermatitis.	Eliminate exacerbating factors, treat noninflamed lesions with emollients, and reserve topical corticosteroids and topical calcineurin inhibitors for inflamed lesions
Name some common exacerbating factors of atopic dermatitis.	Excessive bathing; Xerosis; Environments with low humidity; Emotional stress
When considering treating atopic dermatitis with emollients, what is the optimal vehicle for the topical therapy?	Ointments (petroleum jelly) with zero water content followed by thick creams (Eucerin, Cetaphil) with low water content
Which areas of the body should not be treated with potent topical corticosteroids?	Thin skin of the face and skin folds (can cause irreversible skin atrophy)

PSORIASIS

Describe the most common primary lesion of psoriasis.	Well-demarcated, pink plaques with silvery scale

Describe the primary components in the pathogenesis of psoriasis.

Psoriasis results from hyperproliferation and abnormal differentiation in the epidermis with concomitant inflammatory cell infiltrates and vascular changes

True or false: Psoriasis can be hereditary.

True

Name five different types of psoriasis.

1. Plaque
2. Guttate
3. Pustular
4. Inverse
5. Nail

Name the characteristic signs of the following types of psoriasis.

    Plaque

Erythematous plaques with silver scale on scalp, extensor elbows, knees, and back

    Guttate

Multiple, <1 cm psoriatic lesions on the trunk classically after strep infection

    Pustular

Sheets of superficial pustules and erosions with fever

    Inverse

Lesions in the inguinal, perineal, axillary, and inframammary regions

    Nail

Pitting in the nail plate and with an oil drop sign

Approximately what percentage of patients with psoriasis also have psoriatic arthritis?

30%

Name three classes of drugs that can exacerbate existing psoriasis or result in psoriatic drug eruptions.

1. Beta-blockers
2. Antimalarials
3. Lithium

When evaluating a cryptic rash, involvement in which areas of the body should raise your suspicion for psoriasis?

The presence of lesions in the scalp, umbilicus, intergluteal cleft, and nail plate

What is Koebner's phenomenon?

The development of psoriasis in areas exposed to physical trauma

What is the Auspitz sign?

Presence of bleeding within the psoriatic lesion upon removal of scales

Is there a cure for psoriasis?

No

Name some treatment options for mild, localized plaque psoriasis.

Emollients; Topical corticosteroids; Topical retinoids; Calcipotriene; Classical tar

What type of therapy should be considered in widespread psoriasis?	Phototherapy with ultraviolet light, oral retinoids, methotrexate, and immunomodulatory drugs (such as etanercept, efalizumab)

ACNE

What is the most common cutaneous disorder in the United States?	Acne, most commonly acne vulgaris
Acne is characterized by inflammation of what type of tissue?	Pilosebaceous units of face and upper trunk
Who gets acne?	Can affect all ages, but peaks in adolescence and males can have more severe cases
What are the primary causes of acne?	Increased sebum production; Presence of the bacteria *Propionibacterium acnes*; Abnormal follicular keratinization; Inflammation
Is acne caused by chocolate and fatty foods?	No
Can stress cause acne exacerbations?	Yes
What medications can be associated with acne exacerbations?	Lithium; Hydantoin; Glucocorticoids; Some oral contraceptives; Androgens
What is concerning about a patient with persistent acne and hirsutism?	Possibility of hyperandrogenism secondary to polycystic ovarian syndrome (PCOS) or other endocrine abnormalities
What does acne look like?	Open comedones (blackheads) or closed comedones (whitehead), with papules, pustules, and cysts with or without inflammation
What are comedones?	Keratin plugs forming within the follicular openings
Where on the body does acne most commonly occur?	Face; Neck; Upper arms; Chest; Back
What are topical treatments for acne vulgaris?	Topical antibiotics (clindamycin and erythromycin); Benzoyl peroxide gels; Topical retinoids (tretinoin)
What can be used for more severe acne?	Oral antibiotics (minocycline, tetracycline, erythromycin, and

doxycycline); Isotretinoin for severe, recalcitrant acne

What is isotretinoin?

A 13-cis retinoic acid that is a highly effective oral treatment for acne

What are the indications for isotretinoin therapy?

Recalcitrant acne (less than 50% improvement after six months of therapy with combined oral and topical antibiotics); Scarring acne; Acne with undue psychological distress; Gram-negative folliculitis, inflammatory rosacea, pyoderma faciale, acne fulminans, and hidradenitis suppurativa

What group of people should never receive isotretinoin therapy?

Female who is pregnant or not on birth control, since it is a severe teratogen. The iPledge program has restricted access to isotretinoin

What is the name for the chronic skin disease of the facial pilosebaceous units leading to flushing, telangiectasia, follicular papules, and in more severe cases, lymphedema and rhinophyma (enlarged nose)?

Acne rosacea

Who gets rosacea?

The age of onset is between 30 years and 50 years; females > males

Are acne vulgaris and acne rosacea related?

No. But they can coexist. Rosacea has *no* comedones

What is the treatment for rosacea?

Avoiding trigger factors that cause flushing such as hot beverages, alcohol, UV light, and stress; Topical and oral antibiotics (metronidazole, tetracycline, minocycline); Isotretinoin for severe disease; Surgery for rhinophyma

HERPES ZOSTER

What is the name for the reactivated form of varicella-zoster virus from sensory ganglia?

Herpes Zoster (shingles)

What does herpes zoster look like?

Grouped clear vesicles on an erythematous base occurring in a unilateral, dermatomal distribution

Where does herpes zoster most commonly occur?	Trunk, followed by the head
Who is at risk for herpes zoster?	History of varicella; Age >50 years; The immunocompromised
How common is herpes zoster?	More than 500,000 cases of shingles annually with a cumulative lifetime incidence of 10–20%
How does herpes zoster present?	Prodromal (2–3 weeks): stabbing/pricking pain in the involved dermatome; Acute (3–7 days): new crops of lesions continue to appear for one week progressing from papules → vesicles → pustules → crusts; Chronic (months–years): post-herpetic neuralgia usually resolving spontaneously in 12 months
What is post-herpetic neuralgia (PHN)?	Pain after the skin lesions have resolved
What percentage of patients develop PHN after a herpes zoster episode?	10–15%. Incidence increases with age
How long can PHN last?	Weeks to years
How is herpes zoster diagnosed?	Clinical findings (Tzanck smear, viral culture, or direct fluorescent antibody test can be confirmatory)
What is a Tzanck smear?	A scalpel is used to scrape the base of a fresh blister and then spread on a glass slide and stained with Giemsa or Wright's stain to look for typical multinucleated giant cells
Can herpes zoster be spread?	No. Since it is a reactivation of varicella-zoster virus (VZV), but transmission of primary varicella from an active cutaneous lesion to a susceptible individual can occur
What is the treatment of herpes zoster?	Acyclovir initiated 72 hours after acute vesiculation; Pain control with analgesics, gabapentin, or TCAs

CELLULITIS

What is cellulitis?	An acute infection of dermal and subcutaneous tissue characterized by red, warm, tender skin

What organisms most commonly cause cellulitis?	*Staphylococcus aureus* and *Streptococci pyogenes*
What part of the body is most commonly affected in cellulitis?	Lower legs
A young, otherwise healthy person presents with cellulitis of the arm. What should you suspect?	IV drug use
What should you think of in a patient with bilateral lower leg cellulitis?	Venous stasis dermatitis
How do you diagnose cellulitis?	Clinical appearance
What are some predisposing factors to cellulitis?	Disruption of the skin barrier; Venous or lymphatic compromise; Decreased immunity; A previous history of cellulitis
What is the treatment of cellulitis?	Initial empiric therapy with a penicillinase-resistant semisynthetic penicillin or a first-generation cephalosporin (vancomycin in severe infections or in areas with high incidence of methicillin-resistant *S. aureus*); Surgical intervention with debridement for severe infections

WARTS

What are warts?	A benign epithelial hyperplasia caused by epidermal infection with human papillomavirus (HPV)
What do they look like?	Flesh-colored, hyperkeratotic papules with vegetations, especially on the fingers and extremities
Who gets cutaneous warts?	Anyone is susceptible, but most common in children and young adults
Who is at higher risk for the development of cutaneous warts?	Individuals with decreased cell-mediated immunity and specific occupations (i.e., butchers, meat packers, and fish handlers)
How are warts transmitted?	A break within the stratum corneum allows penetration of the HPV virus through contact with humans or animals infected with HPV

Can they be prevented?	A vaccine for HPV is now available for common serotypes (6, 11) of genital warts
What is the pathognomonic finding for warts?	Black dots within the lesion, commonly referred to as "seeds," representing thrombosed capillary loops
How long do they last?	Resolve in two years in about two-thirds of patients, but may persist for several years
What is the treatment?	Salicylic acid; Cryotherapy; Electrosurgery; Cantharidin; Podophyllin; Imiquimod; Bleomycin; 5-fluorouracil; Curettage and dessication; Cimetidine or duct tape
What location is typically difficult to treat when a wart is present?	Nail beds

SKIN CANCERS

What does the sun protection factor (SPF) indicate?	Measures the time a product protects the skin against burning; if you burn after ten minutes without protection, then wearing sunscreen of SPF 15 will theoretically allow you to stay in the sun 15 times longer before burning
According to the American Cancer Society, how should people protect their skin from the sun when outside?	Use sunscreen of SPF 15 or greater, wear hats, wear shirts and pants when possible, and avoid being outside between 10 AM to 4 PM
How long before sun exposure should patients start applying sunscreen?	30 minutes
What is the most common form of skin cancer?	Basal cell carcinoma (BCC)
What are the risk factors for BCC?	UV exposure; Individual susceptibility; Arsenic ingestion; Previous radiotherapy; Fair skin; Basal cell nevus syndrome; Xeroderma pigmentosum
What are the subtypes of BCC?	Nodular-ulcerated; Superficial; Sclerosing; Cystic; Linear; Micronodular

What is the most common subtype of BCC?	Nodular-ulcerated (about 60% of BCC)
Where does it typically present?	On the face
What is the second most common subtype of BCC?	Superficial (about 30% of BCC)
Where does it typically present?	On the trunk
What is the most common presentation of a BCC?	Shiny, pearly or translucent nodule with telangiectasia, especially in a fair-skinned individual
In what age group does the incidence of BCC peak?	60–70-year olds
What are less common presentations of BCC?	Sore that won't heal; Red, itchy patch; Elevated area with crusting; Waxy area with tight, shiny skin
What are the treatment options for BCCs?	95% can be cured by simple excision or curettage and electrodesiccation. Recurrent lesions treat with Mohs' micrographic surgery. Imiquimod topical cream is also used
An African American male presents with a painless, dark brown discoloration under his toenail and on the sole of his foot, complaining that it has been spreading over the past few months. What is the most likely diagnosis?	Acral lentiginous melanoma
A scaly, crusted, "sandpaper-like" slightly elevated spot on sun-exposed skin that has appeared and disappeared and now reappeared in a 65-year-old male is most likely what lesion?	Actinic keratosis (AK)
What percentage of cases of actinic keratosis progress on to squamous cell carcinoma?	5%
What is the name and implications of an actinic keratosis on the lip?	Actinic cheilitis can develop into aggressive squamous cell cancer
What is the treatment of actinic keratosis?	Curettage; Liquid nitrogen; Topical 5-fluorouracil for 3–4 weeks; Trichloracetic acid
An open sore that will not heal is most characteristic of what form of skin cancer?	Squamous cell carcinoma (SCC)
True or False: Both ultraviolet A (UVA) and ultraviolet B (UVB) radiation from sun exposure increase the risk of SCC.	True

Which type of ultraviolet light is emitted in tanning beds?	UVA
What are some of the risk factors for the development of SCC?	Chronic sun exposure; Individual susceptibility; Skin damage from burns, radiation, chronic irritation, or chemicals
What is the treatment of SCC?	Curettage and desiccation if <1cm; Excision with frozen section control; Mohs' surgery; Radiotherapy
What is the name of the SCC variant that consists of scaly, localized, slow-growing plaques associated with an increased risk of internal malignancy?	Bowen's disease
What does "ABCDE" stand for?	Asymmetry; Border irregularity; Color variegation; Diameter >6 mm; Enlargement or Elevation
What is the ABCDE criteria used for?	Melanomas are highly suspected if a skin lesion fulfills one of the criteria
What are the four types of melanoma?	1. Superficial spreading 2. Acral lentiginous 3. Nodular 4. Lentigo maligna
Which type is most likely to penetrate deep making metastasis more likely?	Nodular melanoma
What is the most common form of melanoma?	Superficial spreading melanoma (70%)
Where on the body are most melanomas found?	Trunk and legs
What is the major determinant of prognosis in melanoma?	Level of invasion (Clark's level or Breslow's thickness)
What is the treatment of melanoma?	Excision; Sentinel node biopsy if more than 1 mm deep; Chemotherapy if metastatic
What follow-up is needed after diagnosis of any type of skin cancer?	Check for development of new lesions every 3–6 months

CHAPTER 10

Rheumatology

RHEUMATOID ARTHRITIS

What is the pathogenesis of rheumatoid arthritis (RA)?
Autoimmune disorder involving chronic inflammation of the synovial lining of joints and destruction of the surrounding joint architecture

RA typically affects what gender and age group of patients?
Females between 30 years and 55 years old

How does a patient with RA present?
Pain and swelling of the hands and feet; Fatigue; Morning stiffness; Fever; Weight loss; Depression

What are the most common joints involved in RA?
Metacarpophalangeal (MCP) and proximal interphalangeal (PIP) joints of the fingers; Interphalangeal (IP) joints of the thumbs; Wrists; Metatarsophalangeal (MTP) joints of the toes

Is the typical joint distribution in RA symmetric or asymmetric?
Symmetric

What criteria are used in the diagnosis of RA?
Four of the following seven criteria must be satisfied for diagnosis:

1. Morning stiffness for six weeks
2. Arthritis of three or more joint areas simultaneously for six weeks
3. Arthritis of hand joints for six weeks
4. Symmetric arthritis
5. Rheumatoid nodules
6. Serum rheumatoid factor
7. Characteristic radiographic changes in the hands

How does a joint affected by RA look on x-ray?
Joint space narrowing and bony erosions

What is rheumatoid factor (RF)?	An autoantibody with specificity to the Fc fragment of IgG
What percentage of patients with RA are RF positive?	85%
Is RF specific for RA?	A high titer of IgM RF is relatively specific for RA if used in the setting of appropriate symptoms (but also seen in other connective tissue diseases and chronic infections)
What is morning stiffness?	Pain and difficulty moving joints upon waking in the morning or after periods of inactivity that then typically improves throughout the day and with movement
What are the classic hand deformities associated with chronic RA?	Ulnar deviation of the hands and swan neck or Boutonniere deformities of the fingers
Describe the swan neck deformity.	PIP hyperextension with distal interphalangeal (DIP) flexion
Describe the Boutonniere deformity.	PIP hyperflexion with DIP hyperextension
What are the extra-articular (systemic) manifestations of RA?	Interstitial lung disease; Pericardial effusions; Ocular manifestations
How is disease activity assessed in a patient with chronic RA?	Symptoms; Functional status; Degree of joint and extra-articular involvement; Laboratory tests; Radiographic changes
Are RF titers used for diagnosis, to follow disease activity, or both?	Diagnosis
What laboratory tests are used to follow disease activity (degree of synovial inflammation)?	Erythrocyte sedimentation rate (ESR); C-reactive protein (CRP) levels
What is the goal of treatment of RA patients?	Early identification and treatment of active disease to prevent permanent destruction of joints
Describe the five classes of drugs used for treatment of RA.	
1. Analgesics	Used for pain control but no affect on disease progression
2. Nonsteroidal anti-infammatory drugs (NSAIDs)	Both analgesic and anti-inflammatory properties but no affect on disease outcome

3. Glucocorticoids	Effective relief of joint pain and inflammation with possible delay of joint erosions
4. Disease modifying anti-rheumatic drugs (DMARDs)	Methotrexate is the most common DMARD and is effective in decreasing disease activity (side effects are the limiting factor)
5. Anticytokine therapy	Antitumor necrosis factor alpha-antibody agents (etanercept, infliximab, adalimumab) are the newest treatments and have powerful anti-inflammatory effects (fewer side effects than DMARDs)
What are the side effects of chronic glucocorticoid use?	Cushingoid features; Peptic ulcers; Cataracts; Osteoporosis; Hyperglycemia; Hypertension; Immunosuppression
What are the classic Cushingoid features?	Truncal obesity; Buffalo hump; Moon face; Weight gain
How much calcium and vitamin D should patients on chronic glucocorticoids take to help prevent osteoporosis?	1000–1500 mg of calcium and 400–800 IU of vitamin D daily by diet or supplementation
What is the mechanism of action of methotrexate?	Structural analogue of folic acid that competitively binds to dihydrofolate reductase, impairing DNA/RNA synthesis and decreasing cellular proliferation
What are the side effects of methotrexate use?	Hepatotoxicity; Pulmonary toxicity (obtain a baseline CXR); Myelosuppression; Nephrotoxicity (from precipitated methotrexate crystals)
If a patient is on methotrexate, how often should you check liver function tests (LFT)?	Every 4–8 weeks
If a patient in on methotrexate, how do you monitor for and help prevent myelosuppression?	Complete blood count (CBC) every 4–8 weeks and prescribe folic acid 1 mg PO daily

GOUT

What is the pathogenesis of gout?	Gout results from the deposition of monosodium urate crystals in tissues or supersaturation of the extracellular fluids

What is the relationship between hyperuricemia and gout?	All patients who develop gout have hyperuricemia at some point in their disease
Will all patients with hyperuricemia develop gout?	No
Who is at highest risk for developing gout?	Men between the age of 30 and 50; Who are obese; Hypertensive; Drink alcohol
What medications can lead to increased uric acid levels?	Thiazide diuretics; Loop diuretics; Aspirin
What are the three clinical stages in classical gout?	1. Asymptomatic hyperuricemia 2. Acute intermittent gout 3. Chronic tophaceous gout
Which joint is most commonly affected in this disease?	First MTP joint (i.e., podagra)
What are the symptoms of an acute gouty attack?	Intensely painful, warm, red, swollen joint that is extremely tender to the touch
What common urologic condition can someone with gout develop?	Uric acid kidney stones
Describe the time-course of an acute gouty attack.	Inflammation reaches its peak intensity within several hours, and resolves within a few days to weeks
What is a brief differential diagnosis of an acute gout attack?	Pseudogout; Acute septic arthritis; Bacterial cellulitis; Traumatic injury to joint
What is the only definitive diagnostic test for gout?	Aspiration of synovial fluid from the affected joint or tophaceous material and visualization of monosodium urate crystals under polarized microscopy
What do monosodium urate crystals look like?	Needle- or rod-shaped, negatively birefringent (under compensated polarized microscopy); Yellow when parallel to the axis of slow vibration
What is the first line of treatment for an acute gouty attack?	NSAIDs (e.g. indomethacin) starting at a high dose, decreased as tolerated, and stopping treatment 48 hours after the attack resolves
What drug may be used for acute gout which is effective in reducing symptoms, but has limited use because it causes GI toxicity in up to 80% of patients?	Colchicine

What is the mechanism of action of colchicine?	Inhibits microtubule polymerization by binding to microtubule protein subunits and preventing aggregation
What drugs may be used if NSAIDs or colchicine are contraindicated or ineffective?	Corticosteroids (intra-articular or systemic)
What prophylaxis is available for patients with recurrent gout?	Antihyperuricemic or uricosuric agents
What antihyperuricemic agent is commonly used and how does it work?	Allopurinol, a xanthine oxidase inhibitor; decreases the production of uric acid
What uricosuric agent is commonly used and how does it work?	Probenecid; increases the excretion of uric acid
When should you not stop or start these prophylactic medications?	During an acute attack
Uric acid is a waste product from the breakdown of what organic product?	Purines
What food items are high in purines?	Meat (especially organ meats such as liver); Fish (especially herring and mackerel)
Why is maintenance of health weight important for people with gout?	Rapid weight loss or fasting can temporarily raise uric acid levels
True or false: Moderate consumption of alcohol, especially beer, as much as doubles the likelihood of developing gout.	True
What is the progression of untreated gout?	Ten or more years of intermittent gouty attacks develops into chronic tophaceous gout
What is a gouty tophus?	A deposition of uric acid crystals built up in the soft tissue of a gouty joint (often have a chalky, gritty consistency and are cream colored if near the skin surface)

SYSTEMIC LUPUS ERYTHEMATOSUS

What is the pathogenesis of systemic lupus erythematous (SLE)?	SLE is an autoimmune disease in which antibodies are formed to various parts of the cell nucleus
What organ systems are most commonly affected in SLE?	Mucocutaneous (80–90%); Musculoskeletal (75–100%); Renal (50–66%); Neurologic (66%);

	Cardiovascular (25%); Respiratory (30%) systems
Which patient population does SLE most commonly affect?	Women between the ages 15 and 40 (female to male ratio is 6–10 to 1)
What is a common initial presentation of SLE?	Constitutional symptoms (fatigue, myalgias, fever, weight changes) in combination with skin and musculoskeletal involvement (but it is not uncommon for renal or neurologic complaints to predominate)
What are the diagnostic criteria for SLE?	Four of the following eleven criteria must be satisfied for diagnosis: 1. Malar rash (butterfly rash) 2. Discoid rash 3. Photosensitivity 4. Oral ulcers 5. Arthritis 6. Serositis 7. Renal disorder 8. Hematologic disorder 9. Immunologic disorder 10. Neurologic disorder 11. Positive antinuclear antibody (ANA) blood test
What are the common skin manifestations in SLE?	Malar rash; Discoid rash; Alopecia; Ulcers in the mouth, nose, or anogenital area
Describe these skin manifestations.	
Malar rash (butterfly rash)	Acute erythematous; Edematous eruption over the bridge of the nose and onto the cheeks; Often brought on by exposure to sunlight
Discoid rash	Chronic and appears as discrete plaques; Often erythematous, involving the face, ears, neck, and scalp; May have scaling; May involve the follicles
Which joints does SLE commonly affect?	Small joints of the hands (PIPs and MCPs), wrists, and knees
Is the joint distribution more commonly symmetric or asymmetric?	Symmetric
What are the renal manifestations of SLE?	Lupus nephritis

The World Health Organization's five-class system to determine the severity of renal disease in lupus nephritis uses what factors?

Sediment; Amount of proteinuria; Serum creatinine; Blood pressure; Anti-dsDNA status; Complement levels

What does the initial clinical evaluation of renal activity of lupus involve?

Urine dipstick; Urine microscopic evaluation; Plus or minus a baseline 24-hour urine analysis for protein and creatinine

What should be monitored serially to assess renal activity?

Blood pressure and urine protein

Describe the following autoantibodies involved in SLE.

Antinuclear antibody (ANA)

Present in almost 100% of people with SLE, so it is used for diagnosis but not to follow disease activity

Anti-dsDNA

Highly specific for SLE and associated with lupus nephritis, can be used to predict disease flares

Anti-Sm antibodies

Insensitive but highly specific for SLE diagnosis

Anti-histone antibodies

Associated with drug-induced lupus

What medications can cause drug-related lupus?

Chlorpromazine; Hydralazine; Isoniazid; Methyldopa; Minocycline; Procainamide; Quinidine

How are the following commonly used to treat SLE?

NSAIDs

Used to treat musculoskeletal complaints

Corticosteroids

Topically for cutaneous lesions; Intra-articularly for joint manifestations; Orally for systemic disease

Antimalarial agents such as hydroxychloroquine

Well tolerated and commonly used to treat constitutional symptoms, skin manifestations, and musculoskeletal complaints

Cyclophosphamide

Used mainly for renal manifestations

What is the natural history of SLE?

An episodic disorder with periods of acute flares and remission

What is the ten-year survival rate of SLE?

80–90%

What usually causes early mortality?   Renal manifestations

What usually causes late mortality?   Cardiovascular disease

Is the disease curable?   No. But many patients enter long
                                                remissions (ANA may even
                                                disappear)

CHAPTER 11

Musculoskeletal System

SPORTS MEDICINE

What are the key components of the Preparticipation Physical Examination (PPE)?

Cardiovascular—family history, symptom history, pulses, murmurs, and blood pressure

Musculoskeletal—previous injuries and symptomatic areas

When should the PPE optimally be conducted?

Six weeks prior to the beginning of the athletic season

What findings in the PPE necessitate further evaluation?

Symptoms of dizziness, syncope, chest pain, and shortness of breath or palpitations with exercise that would suggest an underlying cardiomyopathy; Family history of sudden cardiac death at early age; History of head or spinal injury; Previous heat illness; Best-corrected vision less than 20/40 in either eye; Physical signs of Marfan syndrome; Any systolic murmur grade 3/6 or louder; Any diastolic murmur

What are contraindications to participation in high-contact sports?

Atlantoaxial instability; Hepatomegaly; Splenomegaly; Functional use of only one kidney; Poorly controlled seizure disorder

What are the symptoms associated with the following grades of concussions?

Grade I

Confusion without amnesia

Grade II

Confusion with amnesia

Grade III

Loss of consciousness

What are the return to play guidelines for an athlete with a first occurrence of the following grades of concussions?

Grade I

Return to play in 20 minutes if asymptomatic

Grade II

Terminate play, return if asymptomatic for one week

Grade III

Transport for evaluation at hospital, return to play four weeks after two consecutive asymptomatic weeks

SOFT TISSUE INJURIES

A 35-year-old female complains of pain on the surface of her heel and inside of her foot, which is worse after sitting or when she begins to walk in the morning. She does high-impact aerobics three times a week, and does not remember when she got her last pair of gym shoes. On examination, her pain increases with passive dorsiflexion. What is the most likely diagnosis?

Plantar Fasciitis

What is the etiology of the above diagnosis?

Inflammation of plantar aponeurosis

What are some common causes of the above diagnosis?

Increasing weekly mileage when running or use of inappropriate footwear

What is the most common site for a thigh hematoma?

Quadriceps

"Pain out of proportion" to the injury is characteristic of what injury?

Compartment syndromes

What are the other characteristic symptoms of a compartment syndrome?

Pain on passive motion of fingers or toes; Pallor; Paresthesias; Absent pulses; Inability to move fingers or toes

What are the causes of acute compartment syndromes?

Fracture; Crush injury; Vascular injury; Drug overdose; Burn; Trauma

What is the treatment for acute compartment syndrome?

Emergent fasciotomy

What groups of patients are often affected by chronic compartment syndromes?

Long-distance runners and new military recruits

What muscle compartments are most commonly affected by compartment syndromes?

Anterior compartment of leg and the volar forearm

A 28-year-old runner presents to your office describing lateral knee pain, especially when running downhill, that goes away at rest. He can hear an occasional pop when he is running. On examination, he is tender to palpation over the lateral femoral condyle, and has pain when hopping with a flexed knee. What is the likely diagnosis?

Iliotibial band (ITB) syndrome

Name the physical examination test used in the evaluation of ITB syndrome described below?

With the patient lying down and knee flexed to 90°, apply pressure to ITB over lateral femoral condyle while extending the knee.

Nobles compression test; Pain at 30° is a positive test

Patient lies on unaffected side with knee and hip flexed. Flex the affected knee to 90° and abduct and hyperextend hip while stabilizing the pelvis. Lower the affected leg as far as possible.

Ober's test

Failure to lower the leg to the level of the table during Ober's test suggests what injury?

Tight ITB

What is the treatment of ITB syndrome?

Physical therapy to improve hamstring and ITB flexibility; Nonsteroid anti-inflammatory drugs (NSAIDs); ice; Modifications to activity

What are some risk factors for ITB tightness?

Repetitive flexion and extension of the knee; Long-distance running or cycling; Genu varum; Excessive foot pronation; Internal tibial rotation

Name the soft tissue injury most commonly associated with the following clinical scenarios?

Caused by forced extension of the wrist by brachioradialis or extensive supination.

Lateral epicondylitis (tennis elbow)

Elbow pain from overuse of flexor pronatus, made worse by wrist flexion.

Medial epicondylitis (golfer's elbow or Little League elbow)

Evagination of synovial lining of knee produces painful swelling in calf, negative Thompson test (test to rule out Achilles tendon rupture), able to stand.

Baker cyst (popliteal cyst)

Pain in hip after a direct blow, pain increases in rotation or with lateral bending.

Iliac crest bone contusion (hip pointer)

ACUTE SPRAINS AND STRAINS

What is the difference between a sprain and a strain?

Sprain: stretching of a ligament or joint capsule; Strain: partial tear of muscle-tendon unit

What is the typical history reported by a patient with an acute sprain?

Sudden trauma or fall with "pop" or "snap" followed by pain, swelling, ecchymosis, or difficulty weight-bearing

What is the typical history in a patient with a muscle strain?

Sudden stretch on a muscle while it is actively contracting; If severe, can be associated with a "snapping" sensation

What is the treatment for an acute sprain?

PRICE—Protection; Relative rest; Ice; Compression; Elevation

Upper Extremities

What is the injury associated with the following scenario?

Football player presents with a high-riding clavicle, tenderness at acromioclavicular (AC) joint and intact motor and sensory examinations.

AC separation

An older patient describes poorly localized pain with activities such as overhead lifting or throwing a baseball that has slowly worsened over the last year.

Impingement syndrome, often secondary to rotator cuff tendinitis

A teenage softball player hurt her finger while catching a ball yesterday. On examination, she is tender over the distal interphalangeal (DIP), and unable to extend the joint fully, without evidence of fracture.

Ruptured distal extensor tendon at distal phalanx (mallet finger)

A football player hyperextends his fourth right finger while tackling an opposing player during practice today, and now has bruising and tenderness over the entire volar aspect of his finger and cannot flex the DIP.

Avulsion of flexor digitorum profundus (jersey finger)

A patient presents two weeks after a forced flexion injury of the proximal interphalangeal (PIP) joint. He did not see a doctor initially, but now presents with a flexion deformity of his PIP joint., and you suspect a central slip tear (extensor mechanism proximal to PIP).

Boutonniere deformity

What are the muscles of the rotator cuff?

SITS—Supraspinatus; Infraspinatus; Teres minor; Subscapularis

What bones do the muscles of the rotator cuff attach?

They all attach the scapula to the lateral humeral head.

What imaging modality can best identify a rotator cuff injury?

Magnetic resonance imaging (MRI)

What will this imaging modality show?

Swollen tendon or tear in rotator cuff, with rare calcium deposits on radiographs if chronic rotator cuff tendonitis

What is the treatment for a patient with suspected rotator cuff tendonitis?

NSAIDs and refraining from overhand activities, with a subacromial corticosteroid injection if symptoms persist

What fracture is associated with an anterior glenohumeral dislocation?

Posterolateral humeral head fracture

What is the treatment of a mild collateral ligament sprain of the PIP joint, with no fracture on x-ray, and slight laxity?

Buddy taping to adjacent finger for six weeks, NSAIDs for symptomatic relief

Lower Extremities

What are the key musculoskeletal differential diagnoses of acute knee pain?

Anterior cruciate ligament (ACL) tear; Patellar dislocation; Patellar fracture; Lateral cruciate ligament (LCL)/midclavicular line (MCL); Posterior cruciate ligament (PCL); Meniscal tear

What is the knee injury most typical for each history?

Popping sensation at injury, sensation of giving out or locking, effusion and inability of full extension.

Meniscus tear, medial greater than lateral

Female soccer player feels a pop in her knee when she rotated on a planted foot running.

ACL

A 17-year-old football player hit on the lateral side of his leg by the helmet of the tackling player.

MCL

Hard fall while playing basketball on tibial tuberosity with knee flexed; head-on collision with tibia striking dashboard.

PCL

Often referred to as the "unhappy triad" from being clipped from the side in football, soccer, or other contact sport.

ACL; MCL; Medial meniscus tears

What grade ankle sprains do the following descriptions describe?

Minimal swelling, little hemorrhage, minimal decreased range of motion (ROM)

Grade 1

Moderate "goose-egg" swelling, generalized tenderness, some hemorrhage, and decreased ROM

Grade 2

Diffuse swelling, blurring of Achilles margin, hemorrhage, greatly decreased ROM

Grade 3

What is the most common type of ankle sprain, characterized by pain anterior and inferior to the lateral malleolus?

Lateral sprain from an inversion injury, anterior talofibular ligament (ATFL) > posterior talofibular ligament (PTFL) > Calcaneofibular

What additional injury do you need to worry about with a grade 3 ankle sprain?

Lateral malleolus fracture

What is the injury associated with the following scenario?

Middle-aged weekend warrior hears audible pop while jogging, absent plantar flexion in response to Thompson test (with the patient prone, squeeze the gastrocnemius), can't toe stand.

Achilles tendon rupture

35-year-old male, training for marathon, with pain in proximal-medial aspect of calf, with swelling, ecchymosis, and tenderness, can't stand on toes.	Gastrocnemius tear
What is the name for postero-medial tibial pain, brought on by activity, and improved by rest?	Medial tibial stress syndrome (MTSS), often referred to as "shin splints"
What is the cause of MTSS?	Overuse of anterior leg muscles (ankle dorsiflexors), often early in season or after rapidly increasing level of activity
What are the risk factors for the development of MTSS?	Pes planus (flat feet); Rapid growth; Hyperpronation
What is the name for diffuse knee pain associated with abnormal tracking of the patella through normal ROM, often seen in running, basketball, and soccer?	Patellofemoral dysfunction (PFD)
What is the treatment for PFD?	Rest; NSAIDs; Correct the quadriceps imbalance by strengthening the vastus medialis oblique (VMO)
What disease is associated with trauma to an unclosed ossification system, is considered a traction apophysitis of the tibial tubercle, and occurs in boys more than girls commonly ages 9–15?	Osgood-Schlatter disease

FRACTURES AND DISLOCATIONS

What symptoms are suggestive of a fracture in a patient?	Swelling; Pain with movement; Deformity; Functional impairment; Focal bony tenderness
If you suspect a fracture in a patient that also has a laceration of the skin over or near the fracture site, what type of fracture is it?	Open fracture
Name the fracture described by the following descriptions.	
Fracture perpendicular to shaft of bone	Transverse
Fracture line at an angle to the shaft	Oblique
A fracture with more than two fragments	Comminuted
Fracture line crosses the articular cartilage into the joint	Intra-articular

One cortex of the bone buckles without breaking, usually distal radius of ulna, often in kids	Torus
Fracture fragments are out of their usual alignment	Displaced
A gap exists between the proximal and distal segments of the fracture	Distracted
Angular deformity of a bone without a complete fracture	Greenstick
How are growth plate fractures in children classified?	Salter-Harris fractures— I: Physis (growth plate); II: Metaphysis and physis; III: Epiphysis and physis; IV: All three; V: Crush injury to physis
What Salter-Harris fractures require surgical repair to prevent future complications?	Types III, IV, and V
What are the risk factors for fracture nonunion?	Smoking; Infection; Malnutrition; NSAID overuse; Poor immobilization; Fracture location with poor blood supply
What are the four Rs for treatment of fractures?	**R**ecognition; **R**eduction; **R**etention of reduction with a splint, cast, or fixation; **R**ehabilitation
What is the risk of casting a patient directly following an acute fracture?	Affected site can swell, making the cast too tight and risking a vascular or nerve injury or compartment syndrome
What are considerations in the radiographic evaluation of a long bone fracture?	Include views of joints above and below fracture site to look for dislocation; Obtain images in at least two planes at 90° to each other (AP and lateral); Consider views of asymptomatic limb in children where open physes can make it difficult to identify fracture
What orthopedic injuries require immediate consultation?	Fracture with vascular injury: need ultrasound or angiogram to assess; Pelvic ring injuries: risk of damage to superior gluteal artery
What injuries require orthopedic care within six hours of the initial injury?	Hip dislocation; Open fracture; Penetrating joint injury; Compartment syndromes

What is the name for a bony projection without a secondary ossification center, where a muscle attaches?	Apophysis

Upper Extremities

What is the most common type of shoulder dislocation, usually from a fall on an outstretched arm?	Anterior shoulder dislocation
What type of shoulder dislocation is associated with seizures and electrocutions?	Posterior shoulder dislocation
What is the most common carpal fracture in the hand?	Scaphoid fracture
How is the diagnosis of a scaphoid fracture made?	Fracture on radiographs, or clinical suspicion and tenderness in the anatomical snuff box. Radiographs may take 10–14 days to reveal the fracture
What is the treatment of an uncomplicated scaphoid fracture?	Thumb spica cast for 12 weeks
With a distal interphalangeal (DIP) joint fracture, when do you need to use open reduction/internal fixation (ORIF) to avoid degenerative change?	If >30% of the articular surface is involved
What is the most commonly fractured long bone in children?	Clavicle
What is the major risk for an infant with a clavicle fracture at birth?	Brachial nerve palsy
What type of fracture is most typically associated with the following scenarios?	
A child falls on an outstretched hand.	Distal radius fracture (Colles' fracture if with dorsal displacement of distal fragment)
A three-year-old girl refusing to bend her elbow after being lifted by her hand. Radiographs show radial head subluxation.	Nursemaids' elbow
A 24-year-old male punches a wall and fractures his right fifth metacarpal neck	Boxer's fracture

| A female raises her arms in self-defense, and her left arm absorbs the blow of a blunt object. | Ulnar shaft fracture (Nightstick fracture) |

Name the risks and/or complications associated with the following injuries?

Supracondylar fracture of the humerus	Volkmann's ischemic contracture; Brachial artery at risk
Mid-shaft humerus fracture	Risk of injury to radial nerve and resulting wrist drop and loss of thumb abduction
Proximal third scaphoid fracture in hand	Avascular necrosis (AVN)/nonunion due to disruption of blood supply
Boxer's fracture with skin laceration from punching someone in the jaw	Infection with oral pathogens such as Eikenella. Treat with surgical irrigation, debridement, and IV antibiotics
Non-pathologic fracture of proximal humerus	Frozen shoulder (early ROM exercises when pain improves, out of sling early)

| What are four indications of a probable rotator cuff tear? | 1. Supraspinatus weakness
2. Weakness in external rotation
3. Positive impingement sign
4. Advanced age |

Lower Extremities

What is the differential diagnosis of chronic anterior knee pain?	Patellofemoral dysfunction; Osgood-Schlatter disease; Osteochondritis dessicans; Patellar tendonitis; Bursitis; Patellar stress fracture
The day after presenting to the emergency room with a femur fracture, you are called to the room of a patient noted to be confused and short of breath. On examination, the patient is dyspneic and you notice a scattered pin-point rash. What is the most likely diagnosis?	Fat embolism syndrome
What direction is the patella most likely to dislocate?	Lateral >> medial
A nine-year-old boy presents with pain when squatting down to catch the baseball. He has been playing football three days a week and is on a traveling	Osgood-Schlatter disease (OSD)

Little League team that practices two days a week with games on weekends. On examination, there is localized pain at the tibial tubercle. What diagnosis is most likely?

What is the treatment of OSD?

Decrease activity for 1–2 years (most children will grow out of it). Specialized neoprene bracing can provide symptomatic relief

What type of fracture is most typically associated with the following scenarios?

Fracture of the fibula with avulsion of the base of fifth metatarsal

Jones fracture

Pain with activity, abnormal stress with normal bone, commonly in individuals in sports and military recruits

Stress fracture: Metatarsals (50%); Calcaneous (25%); Tibia (20%); Tarsal navicular (<5%, especially in basketball players)

An osteoporotic woman slips, hears a snap, and is unable to bear weight. She reports it is very painful. On examination, you don't notice any swelling, but see that her left lower limb is externally rotated and noticeably shorter than the right. What are you worried about?

High risk of AVN and deep vein thrombosis (DVT) with a femoral neck fracture

In addition to management of her fracture, what additional medical therapy would you recommend?

Anticoagulate to decrease risk of DVT while in the hospital; Bone health evaluation; Appropriate medication prior to discharge (calcium, vitamin D, bisphosphonate)

Name the risks and/or complications associated with the following injuries?

Fifth metatarsal stress fracture

Nonunion of bone fragments

Tibial fracture

Acute compartment syndrome

What is the most common cause of a limp in toddlers?

Infected joint (septic joint, osteomyelitis, toxic synovitis)

What are the most common causes of a limp in adolescents and teens?

Slipped capital femoral epiphysis (SCFE); Juvenile rheumatoid arthritis (JRA); Avascular necrosis of the femoral head (Legg-Calve-Perthes disease)

What is the initial workup for a child that presents with a limp?

Radiographs of affected joint and above and below joint; Complete blood count (CBC); Erythrocyte sedimentation rate (ESR); C-reactive protein (CRP)

A mother brings in her six-year-old son who presents with two months of a painless limp, along with complaints of mild knee pain. On examination, you notice that he has limited internal rotation, and the affected leg appears smaller than the other. What diagnosis do you suspect?	Legg-Calve-Perthes disease
What is the etiology of this disease?	Avascular necrosis of the femoral head of unknown etiology
What is the treatment of this disease?	Observation if mild; Bracing or hip abduction with a Petrie cast if moderate; Osteotomy if severe
What occurs when acute or repetitive microtraumas cause the femoral head to shear off the femoral neck prior to epiphyseal closure, and causes painful abduction and lateral rotation?	SCFE
What are the risk factors for SCFE?	Obesity; Male gender; African American ethnicity; History of hypothyroidism; 10–14 years old
What radiographic views should you order when you suspect a diagnosis of SCFE?	Radiographs of both hips in AP and Frog-Leg lateral to look for posterior and medial displacement of the femoral head
A college sprinter complains of acute posterior proximal leg/gluteal pain after forcible flexion of the hip with the knee extended. What injury are you most concerned about?	Avulsion fracture of ischial tuberosity at proximal attachment of biceps femoris and semitendinosus (Hurdler's injury)
In what activities is a Hurdler's injury most likely to occur?	Acceleration sports such as sprinting, soccer, basketball, and martial arts
What are the Ottawa ankle rules for when to order an ankle radiograph?	Order AP, PA, and mortise view x-ray if pain near the malleoli plus either inability to bear weight for immediately or in the emergency department (ED) for four steps, or tenderness at or within 6 cm above either malleolus
What are the Ottawa guidelines for when a radiograph is needed in the assessment of a knee injury?	Tenderness at head of fibula; Inability to flex to 90°; Isolated tenderness of patella; Inability to bear weight for four steps: Age ≥55 years (Any one of these with knee pain)

What are the Ottawa guidelines for when a radiograph is needed for a foot injury?

Pain in the mid foot and either inability to bear weight for four steps or bone tenderness at navicular or base of fifth metatarsal

What are the limitations of using the Ottawa rules to guide your decision to obtain radiographs of an injured extremity?

Can not be used for children under the age of 18, the pregnant, and if the patient has multiple painful injuries or if the patient has an injury or intoxication that would decrease their ability to follow the test

Improper use of crutches can result in what injuries?

Axillary artery or venous thrombosis; Radial nerve compression neuropathy

What are the guidelines for fitting crutches to a patient?

Length of crutch should be 75% of the patient's height; Position crutch 4–6 in anterior and lateral to little toe; Place handgrips even with the hips, so arm is 30° flexed; Tops of crutches should be **2 in** below the armpits

BURSITIS, SYNOVITIS, AND TENOSYNOVITIS

What injury is associated with the following clinical scenarios?

Pain on repeated kneeling, with palpable area of swelling between patella and tibial tuberosity, often seen in tilers, roofers who work w/o kneepads

Prepatellar bursitis (housemaid's knee)

Runner started running stairs to prepare for upcoming climbing trip. Point tenderness posterior to greater trochanter, pain with resisted abduction, and lateral thigh rotation

Trochanteric bursitis

What are the Kanavel's signs for tenosynovitis?

STEP: Symmetric Swelling of finger; **T**enderness over flexor sheath; **E**xtension of digit is painful; **P**osture of digit is flexed at rest (surgical emergency!)

What is the mechanism of injury for many cases of septic tenosynovitis?

Penetrating trauma or puncture wound, often from dog bite

If you suspect a septic tenosynovitis, what should you do?

Parenteral antibiotics with coverage for *Staphylococcus* and *Streptococcus* and reevaluate in 12 hours; Continue with oral antibiotics for 7–14 days if patient responds

If a patient does not respond to initial antibiotics, or if infection is purulent, what is the next step?

Urgent evaluation for surgical drainage

A patient presents to your office with swelling at the base of their thumb, and pain that is worse when they try to make a fist or move their thumb. She has lost strength in her grip and ROM in her thumb. What is the most likely diagnosis?

De Quervain's tenosynovitis

What tendons are involved in this condition?

Abductor pollicis longus; Extensor brevis

What physical examination test is diagnostic?

Finkelstein test: full flexion of thumb in the palm, then ulnar deviation of the wrist

What group of patients is most commonly affected?

Middle-aged women

What is the treatment?

Thumb spica splint and two-week course of NSAIDs, with corticosteroid injection if no improvement

DEGENERATIVE JOINT DISEASE

What is the most common joint disorder?

Osteoarthritis (OA)

Describe the pathogenesis of OA.

Progressive destruction of articular cartilage by proteolytic enzymes (proteoglycans, glycosaminoglycans); Remodeling of subchondral bone

What are the most common joints involved in localized idiopathic OA?

Weight bearing (knees, hips, cervical, and lumbar spine); Hands (DIPs, PIPs, carpometacarpals [CMCs]); Feet (metatarsophalangeals[MTPs])

What spinal levels are most commonly involved?

C5; T8; L3: Areas of greatest flexibility

At least how many joints must be involved for generalized idiopathic OA?

Three

What are the risk factors associated with idiopathic OA?

Advanced age; Female sex; Obesity

What are some predisposing factors of secondary OA?

Repeated joint stress; Genetic collagen abnormalities; Metabolic and endocrine diseases (hemochromatosis, diabetes mellitus, hypothyroidism); Inflammatory joint diseases; Neuropathic arthropathy

What is the most common symptom of OA?

Dull, achy pain that is aggravated by joint use and relieved with rest. Pain may occur at rest and at night with advanced disease. It is usually localized and asymmetrical

What are key physical examination findings of OA?

Heberden's and Bouchard's nodes; Squared appearance of hand if first CMC joint involved; Osteophytes; Limited movement; Crepitus; Joint effusion; Malalignment in advanced cases

What are osteophytes?

Bony enlargements at joint margins thought to form in response to cartilage degeneration

Heberden's nodes

Osteoarthritic enlargement of DIPs

Bouchard's nodes

Osteoarthritic enlargement of PIPs

What is the most likely findings when evaluating OA?

Rheumatoid factor

Normal, although may be elevated in elderly

ESR

Normal, except in unusual inflammatory variations

Synovial fluid

Predominantly *noninflammatory* (vs. rheumatoid arthritis); Clear color; Viscous fluid; WBC count $<2000/mm^3$

What are the treatment options of OA in terms of:

Lifestyle modifications and conservative management options

Balancing rest and exercise; Physical therapy; Weight loss; Joint protection; Physiotherapy (heat, cold, ultrasound); Orthotics

Pharmacologic options

Acetaminophen and/or tramadol; NSAIDS in combination with GI protecting agent; Intra-articular corticosteroids

Surgical options

Arthroscopic irrigation or synovec-tomy; Arthroplasty; Artificial joints

What are the complications if OA can arise in the patient's:

    Feet

Involvement of MTP may result in hallux valgus (deviation of great toe toward smaller toes—may result in bunion) or hallux rigidities (stiff big toe)

    Knees

Baker cysts: accumulation of synovial fluid along posterior knee; At risk for rupture; Varus angulation ("bow-legged") or valgus ("knock-kneed") secondary to unequal involvement of medial and lateral compartments

    Spine

Spondylosis (osteophytes arising from vertebral bodies) may lead to spinal cord compression/spinal stenosis; Spondylolisthesis (slipping of one vertebral body on another)

What are the key differences distinguishing OA from RA in terms of:

    Stiffness

OA: Morning stiffness, if present, resolves in less than 30 minutes, but may recur with inactivity ("gelling"); More often, stiffness made worse with activity and relieved with rest

RA: Morning stiffness is significant

    Swelling of joints

OA: Hard; Bony

RA: Soft; Tender; Warm

    Typical finger joints involved

OA: DIPs (frequently associated with Heberden's nodes); CMCs of thumbs

RA: PIPs; Metacarpophalangeals (MCPs)

    X-ray findings

OA: Asymmetric narrowing of joint space; Subchondral sclerosis; Marginal osteophyte formation

RA: Erosions; Cysts

What are the key differences distinguishing OA from calcium pyrophosphate crystal deposition disease (CPPD) in terms of:

    Examination of individual joints

Similar

    Joints involved in CPPD

Knees; Wrists; MCPs; Hips; Shoulders; Elbows; Spine

LOWER BACK PAIN

In patients under the age of 50, what is the leading cause of disability?

Lower back pain

What are the risk factors for malignancy associated with lower back pain?

Personal history of cancer; Age >50 years; Pain not relieved by rest or lying down; Pain that worsens at night or wakes patient from sleep; Symptom duration over four weeks; Constitutional symptoms such as fever, night sweats, and weight loss

What is the differential diagnosis of lower back pain?

See Table 11.1

FIBROSITIS, MYALGIAS, ARTHRALGIAS

What is the most common cause of traumatic neck pain?

Motor vehicle accidents

A 40-year-old woman presents to your office with complaints of chronic pain and fatigue over the last year. On examination, she has multiple areas of soft tissue tenderness, but no tenderness at the joints. What is the suspected diagnosis?

Fibromyalgia syndrome (FMS)

What is the American College of Rheumatology criteria for the diagnosis of FMS?

Generalized pain present for more than three months; Pain must involve the left and right sides of the body, be above the waist and below the waist, and involve the axial skeleton; Pain, not just tenderness, at 11 or more of 18 trigger point sites on digital palpation with an approximate force of 4 kg

What other symptoms do patients with FMS often describe?

Sleep disturbance; Short-term memory loss; Fatigue; Depression and anxiety; Migraine or tension headaches; Substernal chest pain; Paresthesias in hands and feet

What tests are diagnostic of FMS?

No radiographs or lab tests are diagnostic—diagnosis is entirely clinical

What is the treatment of FMS?

Reassurance that disease is not life-threatening; Tricyclic anti-depressants such as amitriptyline; NSAIDs for

Table 11.1 The Differential Diagnosis of Lower Back Pain

Diagnosis	Anatomy and mechanism	Patient description	Abnormal tests
Back strain	Stretching or partial tearing of muscle or ligament fibers	Young to middle-aged pt with back ache and spasm; Limited range of motion; Local tenderness	None
Herniated disc	Gelatinous center of disc (nucleus pulposus) protrudes through the disc's fibrocartilaginous outer rim (annulus fibrosus) and through nerve root canal causing impingement	Middle-aged patient with sharp, shooting pain to buttock and leg; Weakness and paresthesias; Asymmetric reflexes	Herniation seen on MRI; Localized by myelography
Spondylolisthesis	Anterior displacement of vertebra	Presents at any age with lordosis; stiff back; Pain in lower back, thighs, and buttocks; Tight hamstrings	XRs show malignant and possible fracture
Spinal stenosis	Narrowing of spinal canal, nerve root canals; Intervertebral foramina secondary to spondylosis	>50 years; "Pins and needles" sensation and shooting pain increased by walking up an incline and decreased by sitting	XRs may show findings consistent with OA/spondylosis
Ankylosing Spondylitis	Chronic inflammation of intervertebral and sacroiliac joints; Vertebrae may fuse	Young adult male with tenderness of SI joints and decreased back flexion	XRs show sacroiliac(SI) joint narrowing and sclerosis, fusion of vertebral bodies appears as "bamboo spine"

Note: Most of these conditions may be treated conservatively: NSAIDS, muscle relaxants, and physical therapy. Surgery is rarely needed. Ankylosing spondylitis would most likely need a referral; treatment options include NSAIDS, sulfasalazine, immuno-suppressive agents, corticosteroids, and tumor necrosis factor (TNF) inhibitors

short course (no corticosteroids or narcotics); Selective serotonin reuptake inhibitor (SSRI) if severe depression; Topical analgesic agents applied to tender points; Stretching, exercise, and weight loss; FMS support group or visit to established FMS clinic

Pain that persists after an original injury and is out of proportion to the initial injury is characteristic of what syndrome?

Complex regional pain syndrome (CRPS)

What is the classification of CRPS?

Type 1(reflex sympathetic dystrophy)—no identifiable nerve lesion (30%); Type 2 (causalgia)—nerve lesion (70%)

Who is commonly affected by CRPS?

Women >> men; Smokers; Individuals between 30 years and 50 years

What are some of the hallmarks of CRPS?

Allodynia; Hyperpathia; Hyperesthesia; Sleep disturbance; Pain described as "burning or throbbing"

What physical examination signs support the diagnosis of CRPS?

Swelling; Hypersensitivity; Contracture; Overly hot or cold; Atrophy of skin and soft tissue

What is the treatment of CRPS?

Physical therapy for ROM; Adaptive modalities; Oral medications; Psychological counseling; Biofeedback

What medications, although not Food and Drug Administration (FDA)-labeled for chronic pain, often help in the treatment of CRPS?

Antidepressants; Anticonvulsants; Calcium-channel blockers

What are appropriate indications for considering an intra-articular corticosteroid injection?

Rheumatoid arthritis; Osteoarthritis; Crystal-induced arthritis; Tenosynovitis and bursitis (especially flexor tenosynovitis, de Quervain tenosynovitis, trochanteric bursitis, lateral epicondylitis, and plantar fasciitis); Entrapment neuropathies

What are the most common local side effects after a corticosteroid injection?

Lipodystrophy; Discomfort; Loss of skin pigmentation; Transient increased pain for 24–48 hours

What injection sites have an increased risk of infection and should be injected judiciously when other treatment options have failed?

Olecranon and prepatellar bursae

What are some of the adverse systemic effects of corticosteroid injections?	Transient serum cortisol suppression; Hyperglycemia

CARPAL TUNNEL SYNDROME

What nerve is entrapped at the wrist in carpal tunnel syndrome (CTS)?	Median nerve
What conditions can precipitate CTS?	Pregnancy; Diabetes mellitus; Thyroid dysfunction; Overuse trauma; Rheumatoid arthritis
What is the differential diagnosis of pain and paresthesias in the wrist?	Arthritis; Cervical radiculopathy at C6; Ulnar neuropathy; Ganglion cyst; Hypothyroidism; Diabetic neuropathy; Flexor carpi radialis tenosynovitis
What group of people does carpal tunnel most often affect?	Middle-aged or pregnant women
Where do patients typically report paresthesias or numbness?	Median nerve distribution: Thumb; Index finger; Long finger; Half of ring finger
What daily tasks will patients with carpal tunnel often complain of trouble with?	Opening jars; Grasping objects; Twisting lids; Driving; Reading
Aside from the wrist, where do patients often report aching in CTS?	Proximal forearm and in some cases to the shoulder
What physical examination findings can suggest a diagnosis of CTS?	Thenar atrophy; Weakness of thenar muscles; Positive Tinel's sign; Positive Phalen test; Positive Durken test
Identify the name of the following clinical tests used in the diagnosis of CTS?	
Have the patients place the wrists in flexion and look for aching or numbness in the median nerve distribution within 60 seconds.	Phalen's maneuver
The examiner uses their thumb to put pressure over the median nerve at the wrist for up to 30 seconds, looking for either pain or numbness in the median nerve distribution.	Durken carpal compression test
The examiner taps over the median nerve at the wrist and looks for tingling in some or all digits in the median nerve distribution.	Tinel's sign

How is the diagnosis of CTS made?

Clinical history and physical examination; Electrophysiologic testing only to confirm if needed

What is the treatment of mild cases of CTS?

Splinting in neutral position at night and as tolerated during the day; NSAIDs; Ergonomic modifications to keyboards if work-related

What are the indications for referral in CTS?

Failed nonsurgical treatment for three months

If conservative treatment fails, what other therapies can be considered?

Corticosteroid injection to carpal canal; Surgical release if refractory symptoms or persistent sensory loss

What is the treatment of CTS in pregnancy?

Splinting or corticosteroid injection (since most cases resolve after delivery)

CHAPTER 12

Ophthalmology

What are the components of an eight-point eye examination?	1. Visual acuity 2. External examination 3. Pupils 4. Extra-ocular movements 5. Visual fields by confrontation 6. Red reflex (especially in kids) 7. Tactile pressure 8. Fundoscopy
What is the name of the chart composed of letters of the English alphabet of varying sizes used to assess visual acuity?	Snellen chart
What does having 20/40 vision mean?	The patient sees at 20 feet what a normal person sees at 40 feet
How do you test a person that cannot read "the big E"?	Finger counting, hand motion, and light detection (The big E is 20/400)
What are the definitions of the following conditions?	
Myopia	Nearsightedness—the image focuses behind the retina
Hyperopia	Farsightedness—the image focuses in front of the retina
Presbyopia	An age-related thickening of the lens of the eye causing a relative inability to accommodate starting around age 40, requiring the use of reading glasses
Astigmatism	Corneal surface is more elliptical than spherical
What are the common causes of acute vision loss?	Corneal edema; Hyphema; Vitreous hemorrhage; Retinal detachment; Macular degeneration; Retinal vascular occlusion; Optic neuritis; Papillitis; Ischemic optic neuropathy; Giant cell arteritis; Trauma; Vascular complications

What are the common causes of chronic vision loss?

Cataracts; Open angle glaucoma; Age-related macular degeneration; Systemic illnesses (diabetes mellitus [DM], hypertension [HTN])

What symptoms associated with a red eye should raise suspicions of a serious ocular condition?

Blurry vision; Severe pain; Photophobia; Colored halos

What signs associated with a red eye should raise suspicions of a serious ocular condition?

Reduced visual acuity; Ciliary flush (injected vessels around cornea); Corneal opacification; Pupillary abnormalities; Elevated intraocular pressure; Proptosis

What are common eyelid disorders which may present with redness?

Blepharitis; Styes; Chalazions

What is a chalazion?

A minimally tender nodule around the lid margin from chronic inflammation of a meibomian gland

What is a stye?

Tender, erythematous nodule that arises acutely from inflammation of hair follicles at lid margin

What do patients typically complain of with a stye?

Wake up in the morning with a red, painful bump at the lid margin

What is the treatment of styes and chalazions?

Warm compresses with the addition of oral antibiotics if secondary bacterial infection

Will styes go away on their own?

Yes. They typically resolve

Will chalazions go away on their own?

Usually. But they may require incision and curettage under local anesthesia if they do not resolve after 3–4 weeks

What is blepharitis?

Inflammation of the eyelid characterized by scaling and redness along the lid margins

What are the underlying causes of blepharitis?

Staphylococcal infection; Scalp seborrhea; Acne rosacea

What is the treatment for blepharitis?

Warm compresses and eyelid margin scrubs in the morning and bedtime; Topical antibiotics; Antidandruff shampoos

What is orbital cellulitis?

Sight-threatening infection of the fat and muscle contained within the bony orbit

What are the symptoms associated with orbital cellulitis?	Pain with movement of the eye; Redness; Swelling; Blurry vision; Double vision
What are the signs of orbital cellulitis?	Edema (especially conjunctival); Erythema; Limitations of eye movement; Vision loss
What is the most common risk factor for orbital cellulitis?	History of sinusitis
What age group is most commonly affected by orbital cellulitis?	Children
What are the most common causative microorganisms?	Streptococci; *S. aureus*; Non-spore forming anaerobes; Mixed infection (often hard to identify)
What is the appropriate workup of a patient with suspected orbital cellulitis?	Prompt imaging of the orbit to determine the extent of inflammation and the presence of orbital or subperiosteal abscesses
What is the treatment of orbital cellulitis?	Start IV broad-spectrum antibiotic; Consider referral for possible orbital surgery
Why is the incidence of orbital cellulitis decreasing?	H. Flu immunization
What are xanthomas?	Painless, yellowish nodules often occurring on the eyelids as a result of hyperlipidemia
What is dacryocystitis?	Swelling, tenderness, and warmth over the nasal aspect of the lower lid from acute inflammation of the lacrimal sac
How can you make the diagnosis?	Apply pressure to the lacrimal sac to extrude purulent discharge through the tear duct
What is the treatment?	Warm compresses; Massage of the lacrimal sac; Antibiotic ointments
Diffuse redness, irritation, and burning without a history of trauma and often with flu-like symptoms suggest what process?	Conjunctivitis
What are the etiologies of conjunctivitis?	Bacterial; Viral; Chemical; Allergic
A 15-year-old boy with asthma, eczema, and seasonal rhinitis presents with *itchy*, watery eyes. What is the most likely diagnosis?	Allergic conjunctivitis

What is the definitive way to distinguish between bacterial and viral conjunctivitis?

Culture

Although not always reliable, what examination findings might you expect in bacterial and viral conjunctivitis?

Bacterial: purulent discharge, eyes sticking together in morning; Viral: watery discharge throughout the day

What is the treatment of bacterial conjunctivitis?

Antibiotic eye drops 4–6 times a day; Frequent hand washing to prevent spread

Hyperacute onset of profuse, purulent discharge accompanied by intense hyperemia of conjunctiva suggests what process?

Acute gonococcal conjunctivitis

What is the treatment of acute gonococcal conjunctivitis?

Hospitalize with close monitoring; Systemic antibiotics; +/– topical therapy; Frequent eye irrigation

What is the most common cause of neonatal conjunctivitis?

Chlamydia (transmission during passage in birth canal)

How do neonatal chlamydial infections typically present?

Mucopurulent discharge 5–19 days after discharge

How prophylactic antibiotics are given to newborns at birth to decrease the risk of neonatal conjunctivitis?

Erythromycin or tetracycline ointment on eyes

What is the treatment of chlamydial conjunctivitis?

Topical tetracycline and oral erythromycin

What is the typical presentation of neonatal gonococcal conjunctivitis?

Profuse, purulent discharge and striking hyperemia and edema 1–3 days after birth

What is the treatment?

Topical and systemic antibiotics (penicillin, ceftriaxone, or azithromycin)

What should you suspect in a school-aged child who presents with features of gonococcal conjunctivitis?

Sexual abuse

In zoster, what dermatome would have to be affected to affect the patient's vision?

The frontal branch of the first division of the trigeminal nerve (VI)

What clinical examination finding would make you suspect zoster involvement of the frontal branch of VI?

Vesicles approaching the tip of the nose

A 50-year-old white male presents with a wedge-shaped growth on the conjunctiva, extending from the nasal aspect onto the cornea. What is the most likely diagnosis?

Pterygium

What is the treatment?	No treatment unless vision compromised or cosmetically desired
What are the common mechanisms of corneal injury?	Trauma; Infection; Contact lenses worn for long periods; Excessive exposure to ultraviolet light
What is the treatment of corneal abrasions?	Prescribe antibiotic eye drops
What is the treatment of contact lens syndrome?	Topical antibiotics; Analgesics; Artificial tears
What precautions need to be taken in a patient with Bell's palsy?	Protective glasses; Saline eye drops every hour; Lubricant moisturizer with eye taped closed at night
An elderly patient comes in complaining of trouble reading road signs, difficulty driving at night, bothersome glare, and halos around lights. What is the diagnosis?	Age-related cataracts
What are the risk factors for cataracts?	Age; Smoking; Alcohol use; Sunlight exposure; DM; Systemic corticosteroid use; Ocular trauma; Uveitis; Orbital or intraocular radiation
What are the eye examination findings of a cataract?	Darkening of the red reflex; A change in the quality of the red reflex; Difficulty visualizing the fundus using direct ophthalmoscopy
What are the two major systemic diseases that affect the retinal vasculature?	Hypertension and diabetes
What is the treatment of hypertensive retinopathy?	Long-term control of systemic blood pressure
What is the leading cause of blindness in patients aged 20–64 in the United States?	Diabetic retinopathy
Describe the pathophysiology of diabetic retinopathy.	Prolonged hyperglycemia causes vascular endothelial damage and neovascularization
What is the most effective way to prevent or slow the progression of diabetic retinopathy?	Intensive glycemic control
What are the two major classifications of diabetic retinopathy?	Proliferative and nonproliferative retinopathy
What special precaution should be taken in diabetic women who become pregnant?	Comprehensive eye examination in first trimester to look for worsening diabetic retinopathy

A 45-year-old woman complains of sudden onset flashing lights, followed by a large number of floaters in her right eye. What is the diagnosis?

Acute posterior vitreous detachment (PVD) (immediate ophthalmologic consultation to check for retinal tear)

A patient reporting sudden onset of flashing lights and floaters followed by a dense curtain coming down over one eye likely indicates what problem?

Retinal detachment

What is the leading cause of irreversible central vision loss in patients over 50 years of age in the United States?

Age-related macular degeneration (ARMD)

A 55-year-old male with a history of cardiovascular disease reports the sudden, transient loss of vision in his left eye followed by complete resolution. What is the most likely diagnosis?

Amaurosis fugax. Arterial insufficiency leads to transient vision loss

A patient with sudden, painless onset of vision loss and cherry-red spot on funduscopic examination suggests what diagnosis?

Central retinal artery occlusion (CRAO); **C**herry **R**ed and **O**paque **(CRAO)**

If you suspect CRAO, how should you manage the patient?

Immediate ocular massage and consult an ophthalmologist

What disease process is described as a progressive "tunneling" visual field loss usually associated with an increase in intraocular pressure that compresses the optic nerve over time?

Open-angle glaucoma

What are the risk factors for open-angle glaucoma?

Elevated intraocular pressure; Family history; Advanced age; African American ethnicity; Myopia

What glaucoma medications used to treat open-angle glaucoma decrease the production of aqueous humor?

Alpha-adrenergic agonists; Beta-adrenergic blockers; Carbonic anhydrase inhibitors; Cholinergic agonists

What glaucoma medications used to treat open-angle glaucoma increase the outflow of aqueous humor?

Alpha-adrenergic agonists; Miotics; Epinephrine compounds; Prostaglandins

An elderly lady complains of an abruptly painful, red eye with decreased vision and halos around lights as well as nausea and vomiting. Examination shows intense redness around the cornea with corneal haze and a fixed, unreactive pupil. What is the diagnosis?

Acute angle-closure glaucoma

How do you treat acute angle-closure glaucoma until the ophthalmologist is reached?	Anti-emetic, topical agents to decrease intraocular pressure (alpha-adrenergic agonists, beta-adrenergic blockers, carbonic anhydrase inhibitors, cholinergic agonists)
What is the most likely diagnosis in a patient with ocular pain, photophobia, decreased visual acuity, and corneal redness?	Uveitis
What systemic inflammatory illnesses can cause uveitis?	Ankylosing spondylitis; Reiter's syndrome; Psoriatic arthritis; Inflammatory bowel disease (IBD); Sarcoidosis; Behcet's disease; juvenile rheumatoid arthritis; Multiple sclerosis; Kawasaki disease; Systemic lupus erythematosus (SLE); Systemic vasculitis
What are the most common infectious causes of uveitis in a non-compromised host?	Toxoplasmosis; Cat scratch disease; Syphilis; West Nile virus
What are the most common infectious causes of uveitis in an immunocompromised host?	Cytomegalovirus (CMV); Tuberculosis
A young female who presents with acute eye pain worsened by movement, as well as central vision loss most likely has what syndrome?	Optic neuritis
What neurologic disease is associated with optic neuritis?	Multiple sclerosis
A young female presents with diplopia when looking to the right. Eight months ago, she had an episode of weakness in the left leg, that has since almost resolved. What is the diagnosis?	Internuclear ophthalmoplegia; Multiple sclerosis
A patient presents to the emergency department (ED) complaining of blurry vision which began shortly after a tennis ball struck him in the eye earlier that morning. Examination shows a blood level in the anterior chamber. What is the most likely diagnosis?	Hyphema
What is the appropriate management?	Rule out globe perforation or retinal tear
How do you rule out globe perforation?	Look for any sign of pupillary asymmetry

In cases of suspected corneal abrasion, what is the best method of examination?

Fluorescein dye and wood's lamp

What is the appropriate treatment of corneal lacerations?

Topical antibiotics and a tight patch to keep the eye closed for 2–3 days

What mechanism of injury should alert the physician to a globe puncture (open globe injury)?

Sharp object striking the eye; Pulling an object out of the eye; Striking metal

What is the proper method to safely remove a superficial foreign body?

Apply a topical anesthetic and then irrigate the eye profusely

A patient presents to the ED complaining of double vision after a fight. The patient has difficulty elevating the left eye and the double vision improves when one eye is covered. What is the most likely diagnosis?

Orbital floor fracture (blow-out fracture)

What is the diagnostic workup necessary in a suspected orbital floor fracture?

X-ray or CT with orbital floor views

What are the signs of a severe burn injury to the eye?

A white or opaque cornea and pupillary constriction

What is the first step in the treatment of a chemical burn?

True ocular emergency requiring immediate and copious irrigation of the globe for 15–20 minutes with high-flow water or saline

A misalignment of the eyes noted by an asymmetric light reflection is characteristic of what diagnosis?

Strabismus

A decrease in visual acuity due to misuse or disuse of an eye during early childhood is known as?

Amblyopia

What is leukocoria?

A white pupil seen when evaluating the red reflex

What is the differential diagnosis for leukocoria in a child?

Retinoblastoma (47%); Persistent fetal vasculature; Retinopathy of prematurity; Cataract; Coloboma of the choroids or optic disc; Uveitis; Toxocariasis; Coats' disease; Vitreous hemorrhage; Retinal dysplasia

What ocular problem is a child born before 28 weeks at risk for?

Retinopathy of prematurity

What is the most common intraocular malignancy?

Metastatic carcinoma (breast in women, lung in men)

What is the most common primary intraocular tumor in the United States?

Melanoma

What is the most common primary intraocular tumor worldwide?

Retinoblastoma

What is the most common tumor of the eyelid?

Basal cell carcinoma (85–90%)

OCULAR FINDINGS IN SYSTEMIC DISEASE

Name some common ocular findings for the following systemic diseases.

Graves' disease/hyperthyroidism

Bilateral exophthalmos (may not resolve with treatment)

Anemia

Pale conjunctiva

Multiple sclerosis

Optic neuritis; Internuclear ophthalmoplegia; Uveitis

Sickle cell anemia

Direct ophthalmoscopy shows neovascularization and areas of ischemia

Wilson's disease

Kayser-Fleischer ring (brown copper deposits in the iris)

Name the most likely diagnosis for the following.

A "cherry-red spot" on examination in a child

Storage diseases including Tay-Sachs and Niemann-Pick disease and CRAO

A 40-year-old woman presents with dry eyes and dry mouth

Sicca syndrome (Sjögren's)

A four-year-old girl presents with history of multiple fractures and injuries and blue sclera on examination

Osteogenesis imperfecta

A six-year-old boy with cystic fibrosis, newly immigrated from Russia, presents with trouble seeing in the dark and examination shows rough patches (Bitot's spots) on the conjunctiva

Vitamin A deficiency due to malabsorption

CHAPTER 13

Neurology

HEADACHE

What are the common types of headaches?	Tension headache; Cluster headache; Migraine headache
Which is the most common type of headache?	Tension headache
What are the characteristics of a tension headache?	Extended history of headaches and stress, usually with a feeling of tightness in the frontal or occipital regions
How do you treat a tension headache?	Nonsteroidal anti-inflammatory drugs (NSAIDs)/acetaminophen and stress reduction
Which type of headache is unilateral?	Cluster headache (but do not rule out migraine)
What characterizes a cluster headache?	Unilateral; Tender; Severe
What other symptoms are associated with cluster headaches?	Lacrimation; Rhinorrhea; Conjunctival injection
Answer the following regarding the timing of cluster headaches.	
How long do cluster headaches last?	A few minutes to several hours, but usually 30–45 minutes
When do they occur?	Several times a day or at the same time for several days until the "cluster period" is over
How long is a cluster period?	Usually 4–8 weeks
In what gender are cluster headaches more common?	Males
How do you treat a cluster headache?	Serotonin agonists (sumatriptan); Oxygen supplementation

Describe the history given by a patient with a classic migraine headache.

How and where does it hurt?	Intense pounding pain on one or both sides of the head
Preceding and/or associated symptoms	Photophobia; Nausea; Vomiting; Aura (involves vision changes like seeing flashing lights)
Family history of migraine	Yes

How is a common migraine different from a classic migraine?

There is no aura

In what gender are migraine headaches more common?

Females

What typically decreases the pain associated with migraine headaches?

Being in a dark, quiet room; Sleep

How do you treat a migraine headache prophylactically?

Beta-blockers; Anti-seizure medications; Calcium-channel blockers; Tricyclic antidepressants

Acutely

Serotonin agonists (i.e., triptans); Ergotamine; NSAIDs; Narcotic pain meds (sometimes)

What signs and symptoms help you recognize a headache that is secondary to a brain tumor or intracranial mass?

Headache every day that is worse in the morning; Localizing neurologic symptoms (e.g., isolated cranial nerve palsy); Signs of intracranial hypertension

What are some signs and symptoms of increased intracranial pressure?

Nausea; Vomiting; Mental status changes; Ataxia; Papilledema

What are the most acute and emergent causes of headache?

Subarachnoid hemorrhage (SAH); Meningitis (classic pimp question often stated as, "what is the 'worst headache' of a patient's life?")

What are the most common causes of SAH?

Berry aneurysm rupture; Trauma

What are the signs and symptoms of meningitis?

Severe, throbbing headache associated with neck stiffness; Fever; Nausea; Vomiting; Photophobia

What is Brudzinski's sign?

Passive flexion of the head causes involuntary hip flexion

What is Kernig's sign?

Inability to straighten leg when hips are flexed to 90°

When are these two positive?

When there is irritation of the meninges (i.e., meningitis, subarachnoid hemorrhage)

DIZZINESS

What is dizziness?	A subjective sensation of movement of the head, body, or both. Patients may describe it as spinning, light-headedness, vertigo, imbalance, or a falling sensation
Name some causes of dizziness under the following categories.	
Peripheral vestibular disorders	Benign positional vertigo; Meniere's disease; Acoustic neuroma; Labyrinthitis
Systemic diseases	Cardiovascular disease (i.e., arrhythmias, aortic stenosis); Metabolic abnormalities (i.e., hypoglycemia); Anemia; Infection
Central nervous system diseases	Stroke; Transient ischemic attack (TIA); Multiple sclerosis; Basilar artery migraine; Temporal lobe seizure
Psychosocial causes	Anxiety; Depression; Panic disorder; Drug or alcohol use
What causes benign positional vertigo?	It is caused by a change in head position or movement that inappropriately displaces the otoliths into the semicircular canals. It may be accompanied by nystagmus
What physical examination maneuver do you perform if benign positional vertigo is suspected?	The Hallpike maneuver reproduces the symptoms of vertigo and nystagmus
Describe the Hallpike maneuver.	Patient is rapidly moved from a sitting to a head-hanging position
What is Meniere's disease?	Inner ear problem that causes episodes of vertigo, with associated nausea and vomiting, temporary unilateral hearing loss, tinnitus, and a pressure sensation in the involved ear
How long do the episodes typically last?	Minutes to several hours
What is acute labyrinthitis?	Inflammation of the portion of the inner ear responsible for sensing balance causing vertigo and transient hearing loss

What causes most cases of acute labyrinthitis?	Viral infection of the vestibular nerve
What are common ototoxic medications to look for?	Aspirin; Aminoglycosides; Loop diuretics; Quinine; Cisplatin

STROKE

What is a TIA?	It is a focal neurologic deficit that lasts less than *24 hours* (usually <1 hour) due to ischemia
What are common signs and symptoms of a TIA?	Ipsilateral blindness (amaurosis fugax); Unilateral hemiplegia; Hemiparesis; Weakness
Why is a TIA important to diagnose?	May be a precursor to stroke
What is the most common cause of neurologic disability and the third leading cause of death in the United States?	Stroke
What are the two kinds of strokes?	Ischemic and hemorrhagic
Which type is more common?	Ischemic (about 80%)
What causes an ischemic stroke?	A thrombus or an embolic event
What causes a hemorrhagic stroke?	Intracerebral hemorrhage
What is the most common cause of hemorrhagic stroke?	Hypertension (HTN)
What are other causes of strokes?	Coagulopathy; Septic embolus from endocarditis; Sickle cell disease; Ruptured aneurysm; Arteriovenous malformation; Malignancy
What are the signs and symptoms of stroke?	Severe headache; Vomiting; Mental status changes; Nuchal rigidity; Hemisensory loss; Hemiparesis; Amaurosis fugax; Aphasia; Ataxia
What is the initial imaging study you should order if you suspect a stroke?	CT scan of the head without contrast
Should aspirin be given to a patient with a hemorrhagic stroke?	No
When can thrombolysis with tissue-plasminogen activator (tPA) be used in a patient with a confirmed ischemic stroke?	The patient presents within the first three hours of onset of symptoms and meets strict criteria for its use

What are the contraindications of tPA?	Uncontrolled HTN; Intracranial pathology (bleeding, neoplasm, arteriovenous malformation, etc.); Recent major surgery; Recent serious head trauma; Recent stroke; Seizure at onset of stroke; Recent bleeding or risk of bleeding (heparin within last 48 hours and abnormal partial thromboplastin time (PTT), and platelets <100,000, etc.)

BRAIN TRAUMA

What are the four major types of intracranial hemorrhage?	1. Epidural hematoma 2. Subdural hematoma 3. SAH 4. Intracerebral hemorrhage
What causes an epidural hematoma?	Bleeding from meningeal arteries (classically the middle meningeal artery)
What percent of epidural hematomas are associated with a skull fracture?	85%
What causes a subdural hematoma?	Bleeding from bridging veins between the cortex and venous sinuses
What patient populations are vulnerable to subdural hematomas?	Elderly and alcoholics
How do you recognize an epidural hematoma?	The classic history describes head trauma with loss of consciousness, followed by a lucid interval, and then immediate neurologic deterioration
How do you differentiate between an epidural hematoma and subdural hematoma on CT scan?	An epidural hematoma is lenticular or biconvex in shape, while a subdural hematoma is crescent-shaped
What causes a SAH?	Bleeding between the arachnoid and pia mater, usually secondary to trauma or a berry aneurysm rupture
How do you make a definitive diagnosis of SAH?	Lumbar puncture demonstrating blood or xanthochromia (CT may or may not show blood in the ventricles and surrounding brain and brainstem)

CHAPTER 14

Psychiatry

DEPRESSION

What age group has the highest incidence of depression?	25–34 years
What age group is twice as likely to commit suicide as the general population?	Elderly
What medical problems can cause depressive symptoms?	Thyroid problems; Parkinson's disease; Viral illnesses; Carcinoid syndrome; Cancer (especially pancreatic cancer); Systemic lupus erythematosus (SLE); Cerebrovascular disease
What are some common causes of medication/substance-induced depression?	Alcohol; Beta-blockers; Barbiturates; Steroids; Anticonvulsants; Diuretics; Stimulant withdrawal
What are the symptoms of major depression?	**SIGECAPS**:
	Decreased **S**leep (early morning awakenings common)
	Loss of **I**nterest
	Feelings of **G**uilt
	Loss of **E**nergy
	Decreased **C**oncentration
	Change in **A**ppetite
	Change in **P**sychomotor activity
	Suicidal ideation
In order to diagnose a major depressive episode, how long must a person have a depressed mood (or anhedonia) and at least four of the above symptoms?	Two weeks
What it the name for the presence of memory and cognitive defects in patients with major depression?	Pseudodementia

In what group of people is pseudode-
mentia more common?

Elderly

A subtype of major depressive disorder in
which depressive episodes occur only
during months with fewer daylight hours,
and which is often characterized by irritability, hypersomnia, and carbohydrate
craving is known as what disorder?

Seasonal affective disorder

What therapy are patients with seasonal
affective disorder most likely to
respond to?

Light therapy

Do antidepressants differ in their
effectiveness?

No. They just have different side
effect profiles

What are the most common side effects of
selective serotonin reuptake inhibitors
(SSRIs)?

Headache; Gastrointestinal (GI)
complaints; Sexual dysfunction

What are the most common side effects of
tricyclic antidepressants (TCAs)?

Sedation; Weight gain; Orthostatic
hypotension; Anticholinergic side
effects (dry mouth, urinary retention);
Prolonged QT syndrome

A patient who is on a Monoamine Oxidase
Inhibitor (MAOI) and borrowed some of
her friend's antidepressant medication
presents urgently with autonomic
instability, hyperthermia, and seizures.
What is this called?

Serotonin syndrome

A patient who presents with feeling of
guilt, mild sleep disturbance, visual or
auditory hallucinations of the deceased
person, and weight loss three months after
the loss of a loved one most likely is
experiencing what reaction?

Normal grief (bereavement)

If the above symptoms persisted for more
than a year, or involved suicidal ideation,
what would be your diagnosis?

Abnormal grief (major depression)

What are the symptoms of a manic
episode?

DIG FAST:

Distractibility

Insomnia

Grandiosity

Flight of ideas

Increased goal-directed **A**ctivity

Pressured **S**peech

Thoughts racing

How long does a person need to have a persistently elevated and expansive mood and at least three of the above symptoms that cause functional impairment to diagnose a manic episode?	One week
What percentage of manic patients have psychotic symptoms?	75%
A patient that has had an episode of mania, but does not report any depression carries what diagnosis?	Bipolar I disorder
If the same patient had only had hypomanic episodes, but did admit to a major depressive episode in the past, how would your diagnosis change?	Bipolar II disorder
What is the pharmacologic treatment of Bipolar I/II disorders?	Anticonvulsants (carbamazepine, valproic acid); Atypical antipsychotic; Mood stabilizer (lithium)
What symptoms must you ask about before starting a patient on an anti-depressant?	Manic symptoms
Why?	Antidepressants such as SSRIs can trigger a manic episode in bipolar disorder
How does depression manifest itself differently in children as opposed to adults?	Children often present with irritability instead of depressed mood
What percentage of new mothers experience postpartum depression?	10%
What emergent side effect of trazodone must you warn patients about?	Priapism
What does a person taking an MAOI need to avoid?	Tyramine-rich foods (cheese and wine); Pseudoephedrine (hypertensive crisis); TCAs (hyperpyrexia); Meperidine (serotonin syndrome); SSRIs (serotonin syndrome)
What antidepressant is classically associated with an increased incidence of seizures?	Bupropion
What class of drugs is associated with cardiac dysrhythmias and can be lethal in overdose?	TCAs (Limit quantities of these drugs in potentially suicidal patients)
Why do physicians need to closely monitor a child on an antidepressant?	Antidepressant use is associated with an increased risk of suicidal ideation and suicide-related behaviors in children

What are the indications for electroconvulsive therapy (ECT)?

Unresponsive to pharmacotherapy; Cannot tolerate side effects of pharmacotherapy (elderly); If requiring rapid symptom decrease (high suicidality)

What is the major side effect of ECT?

Retrograde amnesia

ANXIETY

Episodes of palpitations, GI distress, dyspnea, and feelings of impending doom that last 5–10 minutes and are twice as common in females than males are typical of what disorder?

Panic disorder

What is the lifetime prevalence of anxiety disorders?

30% in women and 19% in men

What conditions should be ruled out before treatment of suspected panic attacks?

Angina; Myocardial infarction; Side effects of sympathomimetic drugs; Thyrotoxicosis; Carcinoid syndrome; Pheochromocytoma; Pulmonary embolism

What drugs are used in the acute treatment of anxiety?

Benzodiazepines, then transition to SSRIs

What drugs are considered first-line treatment to prevent panic attacks from recurring?

SSRIs. Benzodiazepines can be added to augment disabling symptoms

If a patient with panic disorder also relays to you that she has stopped going to the grocery store, prefers to shop online as opposed to at the mall, and no longer likes riding in elevators, what is your diagnosis?

Panic disorder with agoraphobia

What type of therapy is often recommended as an adjunct for the treatment of phobias?

Cognitive behavioral therapy (CBT)

Strong, exaggerated, and irrational fears of things such as animals, heights, spiders, or flying are known as what types of phobias?

Specific phobias

Irrational fears of situations that can be embarrassing, such as public speaking, making small talk at parties, or using public restrooms, are known as what type of phobias?

Social phobias (social anxiety disorder)

What is the treatment of specific phobias?	Systematic desensitization and supportive psychotherapy
What is the only medication approved for the treatment of social phobias?	Paroxetine is the only Food and Drug Administration (FDA)-approved SSRI
A young female is distressed because she has had persistent thoughts that she has left her front door unlocked at night and gets up multiple times at night to check if it is locked. She knows this is "crazy," but has been falling asleep during the day due to this behavior. What disorder do you suspect?	Obsessive-compulsive disorder
A person who is described by friends as being obsessed with details, organization, and lists, but who perceives no problems with their behavior most likely has what disorder?	Obsessive-compulsive personality disorder
What medications are considered first-line in the treatment of obsessive-compulsive disorder?	SSRIs (often high doses) or TCAs
What therapy can also be utilized as an adjunct to pharmacotherapy in a patient with obsessive-compulsive disorder?	Exposure and response prevention
A patient who describes himself as a "chronic worrier" and has had persistent, hard to control anxiety for more than six months, along with insomnia and fatigue most likely has what diagnosis?	Generalized anxiety disorder (GAD)
What medications are considered first-line in the treatment of GAD?	Buspirone (or other azaspirones); SSRI; SNRI (all combined with psychotherapy)
Why is the above treatment considered first-line?	Lower side effect profile and lower risk for tolerance than benzodiazepines or TCAs

ATTENTION DEFICIT HYPERACTIVITY DISORDER

What are the *Diagnostic and Statistical Manual of Mental Disorders* (Fourth Edition) *(DSM-IV)* criteria for diagnosis of attention deficit hyperactivity disorder (ADHD)?	At least six symptoms involving inattentiveness, hyperactivity, or both that persist for greater than six months; Onset before age seven; Behavior inconsistent with age and development

What medication is considered first-line in the treatment of ADHD?	Methylphenidate (Ritalin)
What percentage of children with ADHD significantly improve after pharmacologic intervention?	75%
What percentage of children with ADHD continue to exhibit symptoms into adulthood?	20% or more
There is an increased incidence of what disorders in children with ADHD?	Mood disorders; Personality disorders; Conduct disorder; Oppositional defiant disorder

CHEMICAL DEPENDENCE (ALCOHOL AND TOBACCO)

What screening questionnaire is specific for alcohol abuse and dependence?	CAGE
What does CAGE stand for?	Yes to two of the questions suggests abuse or dependence:
	Thought you should **C**ut back
	Felt **A**nnoyed by people criticizing your drinking
	Felt **G**uilty or bad about your drinking
	Had a morning **E**ye-opener
What is the lifetime prevalence of alcohol abuse and dependence?	10–15%
What percentage of alcoholics have a comorbid mental disorder?	50%
What syndrome caused by chronic alcohol use is characterized by abrupt onset encephalopathy, truncal ataxia, confusion, and ophthalmoplegia?	Wernicke's encephalopathy (Reversible)
When this syndrome progresses to confabulation and anterograde amnesia, what is it called?	Korsakoff's syndrome (Irreversible)
What vitamin deficiency is the cause of Wernicke-Korsakoff's syndrome?	Thiamine deficiency
What is the mechanism of disulfiram (Antabuse) in the treatment of alcoholism?	Blocks acetaldehyde dehydrogenase, which prevents the conversion of acetaldehyde to acetic acid, causing acetaldehyde accumulation and

adverse symptoms such as nausea and vomiting

Why do some people experience flushing and nausea after drinking mild amounts of alcohol?

Less acetaldehyde dehydrogenase causes buildup of acetaldehyde

At what Blood Alcohol Level do the following side effects of alcohol consumption appear?

Decreased fine motor control

20–50 mg/dL

Poor balance

100–150 mg/dL

Coma

300 mg/dL

What are the treatment options for alcohol dependence?

Support groups (such as Alcoholics Anonymous); Disulfiram; Naltrexone; psychotherapy; SSRIs

What nutritional supplementation should patients with alcohol dependence receive?

Thiamine; Folic acid; Multivitamins

What is the primary defense mechanism in alcoholics?

Denial

What is the first step in the 12-step program of Alcoholics Anonymous?

"We admitted we were powerless over alcohol and that our lives had become unmanageable."

What fraction of those who try nicotine will become addicted?

One-third

What does the US Public Health Service recommend physicians to use when treating patients with nicotine addictions?

Five As:

Ask about tobacco use at every visit

Advise all smokers to quit

Assess the patient's willingness to quit

Assist the patient in attempt to quit

Arrange follow-up

What are the risks associated with cigarette smoking during pregnancy?

Low birth weight and persistent pulmonary hypertension in the newborn

What are the symptoms of nicotine withdrawal?

Craving; Anxiety; Dysphoria; Increased appetite; Irritability; Insomnia

True or False: A former smoker can reduce their risk of developing coronary heart disease by 50% within one year of quitting.

True

How many times do smokers attempt to quit smoking on average before cessation is successful?	4–5 times
What steps does the "stages of change" model entail?	1. Precontemplation 2. Contemplation 3. Preparation 4. Action 5. Maintenance
What form of nicotine replacement therapy (NRT) seems to be the most effective?	Similar results for the gum, patch, spray, lozenge, and inhaler
What medications are the only non-nicotine therapy FDA-approved for smoking cessation?	Bupropion SR (Zyban) and Varenicline Tartrate (Chantix)
In what groups of patients is Bupropion contraindicated?	Patients with seizure disorders, bulimia, or anorexia nervosa, history of head trauma, currently using an MAOI; Pregnant women
What smoking cessation intervention is often used for smokers who also have high blood pressure?	Clonidine
What smoking cessation intervention is often used for smokers who also have depression?	Nortriptyline

Identify the illegal substance most likely to cause the following effects?

Intense changes in sensory perception and flashbacks	LSD; MDMA
Conjunctival injection, increased appetite, dry mouth, tachycardia, impaired motor coordination, and impaired judgment	Cannabis
Impulsivity, psychomotor agitation, nystagmus, tachycardia, diminished responsiveness to pain, and ataxia	PCP
Euphoria, hypervigilance, anxiety, papillary dilation, diaphoresis, nausea or vomiting, and confusion	Amphetamine
Grandiosity, tachycardia, papillary dilation, psychomotor agitation, formication	Cocaine

Pupillary constriction, drowsiness, slurred speech, euphoria followed by apathy — Heroin; Narcotics

EATING DISORDERS

Body weight at least 15% below normal, intense fear of gaining weight, distorted body image, and amenorrhea are characteristics of what disorder? — Anorexia nervosa

How is the diagnostic weight criteria for anorexia modified to apply to a child or adolescent? — Failure to make expected weight gain during a period of growth

What are the two subtypes of anorexia nervosa? —
1. Restricting type
2. Binge-eating/purging type

What are some of the physical signs of anorexia? — Amenorrhea; Electrolyte abnormalities; Hypotension; Bradycardia; Cardiac arrhythmias; Lanugo (fine body hair); Osteoporosis; Low body temperature; Leukopenia; Melanosis coli (darkened section of colon from laxative abuse)

What are the common causes of mortality in patients with anorexia? — Starvation; Suicide; Electrolyte disturbances

What are the indications for hospitalization for anorexia? — Body weight 20% below ideal body weight

What is the most likely diagnosis in a patient who is overly concerned with body weight and behaviors to prevent weight gain (laxative use or over-exercising), engages in recurrent episodes of binge eating, but maintains a normal body? — Bulimia nervosa

What are the two subtypes of bulimia? —
1. Purging type
2. Non-purging type

What is Russell's sign? — Abrasions on the dorsum of the hand from repeated self-induced vomiting

What are some of the physical signs of bulimia? — Erosive esophagitis; Dental erosion; Russell's sign; Hypertrophic salivary glands; Hypochloremic hypokalemic alkalosis

DOMESTIC VIOLENCE

What disorders are more common in
a patient in an abusive relationship?

Substance abuse; Anxiety;
Depression; Eating disorders

What is a serious long-term consequence
of intimate partner violence?

Post-traumatic stress disorder
(Flashbacks and dissociation are
common)

Victims of abuse often report what
somatic complaints?

Chronic abdominal pain; Headaches;
Fatigue; Chronic pelvic pain

Frequent emergency room visits,
noncompliance, coming late for prenatal
care, and inconsistent injuries can all be
suggestive of what problem?

Abusive relationship in the home

What is a widely recommended screening
tool for domestic violence?

SAFE questions

What does SAFE stand for?

Do you feel **S**afe in your
relationship?

Have you ever been **A**fraid in your
relationship?

Are **F**riends and **F**amily aware?

Do you have an **E**mergency plan?

Does screening for intimate partner
violence decrease disability or premature
death?

No. But many practitioners still
advocate screening

When is reporting of domestic violence
mandatory?

If person is under the age of 18 or
over the age of 60. But six states
mandate reporting for all victims

How can a physician get more information
about domestic violence resources?

1-800-799-SAFE (National Domestic
Violence Hotline)

DELIRIUM AND DEMENTIA

What are some of the differences in the
time course of delirium and dementia?

Delirium: Acute; Transient;
Fluctuating

Dementia: Slower; Often stepwise
downhill progression

Impaired memory and cognitive function
without an alteration in consciousness is
characteristic of what disorder?

Dementia

What percentage of patients older than 80 have a severe form of dementia?	20%
What are the most common causes of dementia?	Alzheimer's dementia (80%); Vascular dementia; Major depression (pseudodementia)
What is the average life-expectancy for a patient with Alzheimer's after initial diagnosis?	Eight years
A fluctuating course with lucid intervals, also known as "waxing and waning" consciousness, is the key to diagnosing what disorder?	Delirium
What are some of the most common causes of delirium?	Systemic illness; Drug abuse or withdrawal; Medication side effects; Cerebrovascular accident (CVA); Central nervous system (CNS) disease; Hypoxia
What is the key to management of delirium?	Treat the underlying cause
What measures can you take to help orient a patient with delirium?	Avoid napping; Keep the lights on and have a window visible during the day; Frequently reorient the patient; 1:1 nursing for safety; Antipsychotics as needed for symptoms of psychosis
What is the technical name for minor forgetfulness that many persons experience as a consequence of normal aging?	Benign senescent forgetfulness

SOMATIZATION

For each of the following scenarios of somatization, what is the most likely diagnosis?	
Conversion disorder	Sensory or motor symptom, often neurologic and preceded by a conflict or stressor that has no findings in the medical workup
Hypochondriasis	Preoccupation with having a serious disease due to misinterpretation of bodily sensations
Factitious disorder	Symptoms intentionally created to assume sick role. Can occur by proxy in children under two (Munchausen syndrome by proxy)

Somatization disorder   Four or more pain symptoms: two GI,
                                   one sexual/reproductive, and one
                                   pseudoneurologic

Malingering   *Conscious*, feigned for secondary
                                   gain, often financial

Pain disorder   Pain in one or more sites that causes
                                   significant distress, not intentional

CHAPTER 15

Genitourinary System

INCONTINENCE

What is urinary incontinence?	Involuntary loss of urine
What are the types of urinary incontinence?	Stress incontinence; Urge incontinence; Neuropathic incontinence (overflow); Mixed incontinence
What is stress incontinence?	Involuntary loss of urine when the intra-abdominal pressure is greater than the pressure generated by the urinary sphincter (coughing, lifting, sneezing)
Who is most commonly affected by stress incontinence?	Middle-aged, multiparous women
What is the underlying pathophysiology of stress incontinence?	Weakness of the pelvic floor and hypermobility of the vesicourethral segment
What are the signs of stress incontinence?	Anterior pelvic prolapse; Cystocele or urethrocele; Positive Marshall test
What is the Marshall test?	With the woman in dorsal lithotomy, fill the bladder and ask her to cough. Women with pelvic floor instability will leak urine
What is the definitive treatment for stress incontinence?	Surgical pelvic floor suspension
What medications are used to treat stress incontinence?	Alpha-adrenergic agonists
What other adjunctive treatments can help stress incontinence?	Mild cases can respond to Kegel exercises to strengthen the pelvic floor musculature or the use of pessaries in females
What is the pathophysiology of urge incontinence?	The detrusor spasms against a functioning urinary sphincter

What are the symptoms of urge incontinence?

The patient complains of the sudden urge to urinate and leaks urine or urinates on the way to the bathroom

What are the common signs?

No findings on physical examination, but will have abnormal urodynamic studies

What medications are used to treat urge incontinence?

Anticholinergic medications (oxybutynin, tolterodine, etc.) to prevent detrusor spasm

What are the common side effects of anticholinergic medications?

Dry mouth; Dizziness; Drowsiness; Constipation; Nausea; Blurry vision

What is an absolute contraindication to anticholinergic therapy?

Uncontrolled narrow angle glaucoma

What is neuropathic incontinence?

Incontinence caused by a lesion of the nervous system (stroke, spinal cord lesion, dementia, Parkinson's)

What is the treatment for neuropathic incontinence?

Intermittent self-catheterization

IMPOTENCE

What is the definition of impotence (erectile dysfunction)?

Inability to initiate, achieve, or maintain an erection sufficient for satisfactory sexual performance

What is the prevalence of erectile dysfunction (ED)?

One-third of men at age 40 and two-thirds of men by the age of 70

What are the common etiologies of ED?

Initiation problems: psychologic, neurologic, and endocrine; Filling problems: arterial; Storage problems: venous or structural occlusion

What are some common risk factors for ED?

Diabetes mellitus; Atherosclerosis; Heart disease; Hypertension; Medications; Previous prostate surgery

What medications can cause ED?

Antihypertensives (especially beta-blockers); Alcohol; H2 antagonists; 5-alpha reductase inhibitors; Aldosterone antagonists; SSRIs

What sexual changes are considered part of normal aging in a male?

Increased time to erection; Increased refractory period; More rapid loss of erection after stimulation

What are the first-line treatments for ED?

PDE-5 inhibitors (sildenafil, vardenafil); Psychotherapy; Sex

therapy; Testosterone injections
(if hypogonadism)

What is the mechanism of PDE-5 inhibitors?

Inhibit phosphodiesterase-5 preventing the degradation of cGMP, which enhances the relaxing effect of nitric oxide on the smooth muscle of the arteries of the penis

What commonly used medication can cause dangerous drops in blood pressure when used with PDE-5 inhibitors?

Nitrates

What treatments can be tried after failure of first-line treatments for ED?

Vacuum pumps; Intracavernosal injections; Implantation of semirigid or inflatable prostheses

Intracavernosal self-injection with papaverine can often cause what serious side effect?

Priapism

A patient with sickle-cell disease should not use what treatment for ED?

Vacuum constriction device (can cause ischemic injury to penis from sickling)

BENIGN PROSTATIC HYPERPLASIA

What is benign prostatic hyperplasia (BPH)?

An enlargement of the prostate considered a normal part of aging in men over the age of 50 that can cause symptoms of urinary obstruction

What is the prevalence of BPH?

25% of men at age 55 and 80% at age 80 report obstructive voiding symptoms

What area of the prostate does BPH most commonly occur?

Central zone. It may not be detected on examination

What is the differential diagnosis for lower urinary tract outlet obstruction in men?

BPH; Urinary tract infection (UTI); Neurogenic bladder; Urethral stricture; Bladder stone; Bladder neck contracture

What are the obstructive symptoms of BPH?

Hesitancy; Decreased stream; Sensation of incomplete voiding; Straining; Post-void dribbling

What are the irritative symptoms of BPH?

Urgency; Frequency; Opening hematuria; Nocturia

What digital rectal examination findings are characteristic of BPH?

Uniform enlargement; Rubbery texture

What digital rectal examination findings would suggest malignancy?	Hard nodules; Irregular texture
What labs should be ordered and why?	Creatinine: rules out obstructive uropathy or renal insufficiency; Urinalysis/urine culture: rules out infection and hematuria
What is the medical treatment of BPH?	Alpha-adrenergic blockers (prazosin, terazosin); 5-alpha reductase inhibitors (finasteride)
What is the surgical treatment of BPH?	Transurethral resection of the prostate (TURP) or open prostatectomy if severe
What is the mechanism of action of alpha-1-adrenergic blockers?	Relax the prostate smooth muscle alleviating the dynamic component of the obstruction and relax the bladder's internal sphincter
What are the common side effects of alpha-1-adrenergic blockers?	Orthostatic hypotension; Retrograde ejaculation
How long does it take these drugs to effect a change in symptoms?	One week
What is the mechanism of action of 5-alpha reductase inhibitors?	Inhibit the conversion of testosterone to the more potent androgen dihydrotestosterone (DHT), resulting in a decrease in the size of the prostate
What are the common side effects of 5-alpha reductase inhibitors?	Decreased libido; Decreased ejaculate volume; Impotence; Gynecomastia
What effect do 5-alpha reductase inhibitors have on prostate specific antigen (PSA)?	Reduce the PSA by 50%
How long does it take for 5-alpha reductase inhibitors to have their full effect?	Six months
What are the indications for surgical intervention in BPH?	Refractory urinary retention; Recurrent UTI from BPH; Recurrent gross hematuria; Bladder stone formation; Renal failure; Large bladder diverticula

PROSTATE CANCER

What cancer is the most common cancer in men and the second leading cause of cancer death in men (after lung cancer)?	Prostate cancer (CaP)

What are the risk factors for CaP?

Advanced age; Positive family history; African American ethnicity; High dietary fat intake

What are the screening guidelines for CaP?

Annual digital rectal examination (DRE) over the age of 50 (40 if African American or with a first-degree relative with a history of prostate cancer)

What findings would suggest a diagnosis of CaP?

Elevated PSA >4 ng/mL with or without symptoms (obstructive symptoms, constitutional symptoms, back pain due to metastasis)

What can cause an elevation in the PSA?

CaP; BPH; Acute prostatitis; Prostate massage; Prostate biopsy

How is CaP definitively diagnosed?

Biopsy

What is the most common indication for a prostate biopsy?

Asymptomatic rise in the PSA without a palpable lesion on digital rectal examination

What is the most common pathology of CaP?

Adenocarcinoma (95%); Transitional cell carcinoma (4.5%); Neuroendocrine or sarcomas (<1%)

Where does CaP usually originate?

Peripheral zone (70%)

How is CaP graded?

The Gleason histologic score.

How do you calculate this?

The pathologists assign a primary grade of 1–5 to the most commonly observed pattern and a secondary grade to the second most common, and then the grades are summed

What are the treatment options for CaP?

Watchful waiting (low-grade lesions or poor treatment candidates); Radical prostatectomy; External beam radiation; Brachytherapy; Cryosurgery; Local radiation (seed implants)

What are the common sites of metastasis?

Osteoblastic bone lesions (most common) or lung; Liver; Adrenal; Obturator and hypogastric nodes

What are the indications for a bone scan in a new diagnosis of prostate cancer?

Patient is complaining of symptoms suspicious for bony metastasis; A PSA >10 ng/mL or elevated serum calcium or alkaline phosphatase on chemistries

What is the treatment for metastatic CaP?   Androgen ablation with LHRH
                                                             agonists and testosterone antagonists
                                                             along with systemic chemotherapy

URINARY TRACT INFECTION

A 25-year-old, previously healthy, sexually   UTI
active female presents with dysuria,
frequency, urgency, and suprapubic pain.
She is afebrile and without flank pain.
What is the most likely diagnosis?

What is the differential diagnosis for the   Vaginitis; Urethritis; STDs; Prostatitis
typical symptoms of a UTI?

A UTI is loosely defined to describe   Urethra (urethritis); Bladder (cystitis);
an infection of what structures?   Prostate (prostatitis); Kidney
                                                             (pyelonephritis)

What symptoms might you also see in   Bed-wetting; Poor feeding; Irritability;
a child with a UTI?   Fevers

What are the four most common   1. *Escherichia coli* (80%)
organisms that cause UTIs in otherwise   2. *Staphylococcus saprophyticus* (10–15%)
healthy persons in the community?   3. *Proteus mirabilis*
                                                             4. *Klebsiella*

What are some of the common risk factors   Sexual activity; Failure to void after
for UTI?   intercourse; Diaphragm and
                                                             spermicide use; Previous UTI; Recent
                                                             antibiotic use; Catheters or urologic
                                                             instrumentation; Obstruction (BPH,
                                                             stones, adhesions); Pregnancy;
                                                             Diabetes; Immunosuppression

If a patient develops a UTI while   *Pseudomonas aeruginosa* and
hospitalized, what other organisms   *Staphylococcus aureus*
should you also consider?

How is the diagnosis of UTI established?   Often diagnosed based on symptoms
                                                             (urinalysis and urine culture in
                                                             failures or uncertain of diagnosis)

What are the findings on urinalysis?   Positive **leukocyte esterase**
                                                             (produced by the breakdown of
                                                             white blood cells in the urine);
                                                             Positive **urinary nitrite** (produced by
                                                             reduction of dietary nitrates by many
                                                             gram-negative bacteria); White blood
                                                             cells and/or red blood cells on
                                                             microscopy

What is the sensitivity and specificity of a positive leukocyte esterase?	75% sensitive, 95% specific
What is the threshold for UTI on quantitative urine culture?	100,000 CFU/mL. (50% of symptomatic infections will have only 1000 CFU/mL)
What group of persons is the only group that should be treated for asymptomatic bacteriuria?	Pregnant women
What antibiotics are used as first-line empirical treatment of an uncomplicated UTI?	Trimethoprim/sulfamethoxazole double-strength tablet PO daily for three days in women, and seven days in men
What antibiotic might you choose for a complicated infection, or in an area with more than 15% trimethoprim/ sulfamethoxazole resistance?	Fluoroquinolones (not in pregnancy)
What antibiotic is commonly used to treat UTI or asymptomatic bacteriuria in pregnancy?	Nitrofurantoin for seven days
What recommendations would you make for a woman who has recurrent urinary tract infections?	Void after intercourse; Antimicrobial prophylaxis daily or 3×/week or after intercourse with nitrofurantoin; Topical estrogen therapy in postmenopausal women
A 30-year-old male presents with frequency and urgency symptoms. He denies fever, chills or flank pain, and does not have any penile discharge. What do you suspect?	Uncomplicated UTI
If the same patient presents with a second infection, or had symptoms of pyelonephritis, what should you do?	Urologic evaluation
What are the risk factors for UTI in a young adult male?	Anal intercourse; Lack of circumcision; Sexual partner with vaginal colonization with *E. coli*

PYELONEPHRITIS

What is pyelonephritis?	Inflammation of the kidney and renal pelvis
What is the classic triad of pyelonephritis?	1. Chills 2. Fever 3. Costovertebral angle tenderness

What percentage of patients with pyelonephritis develop urosepsis?

20–30% of patients

What is the most common etiology of UTI and pyelonephritis?

Ascending infection

What are the causative organisms?

Organisms that **SCEEK PP:**
Serratia
Citrobacter
Enterobacter
Escherichia coli (80%)
Klebsiella
Proteus
Pseudomonas

How is the diagnosis of pyelonephritis made?

Clinical diagnosis supported by lab findings such as urine WBC or WBC casts

What is the only laboratory test that can immediately and specifically support the diagnosis of pyelonephritis?

White cell casts (sign of infection in renal medulla)

What are the symptoms and signs of pyelonephritis?

Fever; Flank pain; Nausea; Vomiting; Costovertebral angle tenderness; Urgency; Frequency; Dysuria

Pain in the loin on deep percussion of the kidneys over the costovertebral angle is also known as what sign?

Lloyd's sign

Are imaging studies such as CT or ultrasound helpful in establishing the diagnosis of pyelonephritis?

No

What are the indications for hospitalization in pyelonephritis?

Inability to tolerate oral hydration and medications; Noncompliance with medical treatment; Severe illness; Pregnancy; Other comorbid conditions; Area of high resistance to antibiotics

What is the appropriate antibiotic treatment for pyelonephritis?

Start with an aminoglycoside, quinolone, or third-generation cephalosporin. Change your antibiotic as needed, depending on the urine culture results. Treat for 14 days total.

CHAPTER 16

Women's Health

CERVICAL CANCER

What are the soft, fleshy exophytic genital warts caused by human papillomavirus (HPV) called?	Condyloma accuminata
How can HPV warts be treated?	Excision; Liquid nitrogen; Podophyllin solution; Imiquimod cream
Which HPV serotypes cause 90% of cases of genital warts?	6 and 11
What is the biggest risk factor for developing cervical dysplasia and cancer?	HPV infection
Which HPV serotypes cause 70% of cases of cervical cancer?	16 and 18
Which HPV serotypes are considered "high-risk" for causing cervical cancer?	16, 18, 31, 33, 35, 39, 45, 51, 52, 56, 58, 59, 68, 69
What is the transformation zone?	The area between the old and new squamocolumnar junction, where squamous metaplasia commonly occurs
What other factors may place a woman at higher risk for cervical dysplasia?	Early intercourse; Multiple sex partners; Early childbearing; History of sexually transmitted infections; Immunocompromised; Oral contraceptive pills (OCP) use; Smoking; Intrauterine diethylstilbestrol (DES) exposure
What are the current recommendations for when to initiate Pap screening (per the American College of Obstetricians and Gynecologists [ACOG])?	First Pap smear three years after first sexual intercourse or at age 21, whichever comes first
By how much does annual Pap screening decrease the incidence of invasive cervical cancer?	More than 95%

The following questions are about
when women can stop getting annual
Pap smears.

True or False: Women ≥30 years with   True
three consecutive negative Paps, no
history of cervical intraepithelial
neoplasia (CIN) II/III, who are not
immunocompromised and were not
exposed to DES in utero may get Pap
smears every three years.

True or False: Women who have   True
undergone hysterectomy with removal
of the cervix for benign indications and
who have no prior history of CIN II/III
or worse may discontinue routine Pap
smears.

At what age may women discontinue   American Cancer Society
getting Pap smears altogether?   recommends age 70 and the United
                                             States Preventive Services Task Force
                                             (USPSTF) recommends age 65 if
                                             adequate previous screening was
                                             done, and the patient is low-risk

What are the cytologic classifications of   ASCUS (atypical squamous cells of
abnormal Pap smears?   undetermined significance); ASC-H
                                             (atypical squamous cells suspicious
                                             of high-grade intraepithelial lesions);
                                             LSIL (low-grade squamous
                                             intraepithelial lesions); HSIL (high-
                                             grade squamous intraepithelial
                                             lesions)

What are the pre-cancerous histologic   CIN I (dysplasia confined to the
classifications of abnormal Pap smears?   basal one-third of the epithelium);
                                             CIN II (dysplasia confined to the
                                             basal two-thirds of the epithelium);
                                             CIN III (dysplasia of more than two-
                                             thirds of the epithelium)

What is colposcopy?   A technique used to evaluate cervical
                                             dysplasia that involves a special
                                             microscope to visualize the cervix

Fill in the blank: During colposcopy, ____   Acetic
acid can be applied to the cervix in order
to visualize the abnormal areas of the
epithelium (area turns white).

What other chemicals can be placed on the   Lugol's or Schiller's iodine solution
cervix during colposcopy for visualization
of lesions?

What procedures can be performed along with colposcopy?	Cervical biopsies and endometrial curettage
What options are available for the management of atypical squamous cell of uncertain significance (ASC-US)?	Triage to colposcopy based on HPV testing; Accelerated serial cytology smears; Immediate referral to colposcopy
Describe the management of a patient with ASC-US and the following HPV testing results.	
High-risk types of HPV DNA	Colposcopy immediately
Negative high-risk HPV DNA	Repeat Pap in 12 months
What is the management of ASC-US based on accelerated serial cytology smears?	Repeat the smear in six months
What do you do if the repeat smear is normal?	Repeat accelerated smears (every six months) until two consecutive normal smears, and then resume routine screening
What do you do if the repeat smear is abnormal (ASC-US or greater)?	Colposcopy
What is the initial management of LSIL and HSIL?	Immediate colposcopy
What is the risk of CIN II/III with LSIL?	15–30%
What is the risk of CIN II/III with HSIL?	70–75%
How is cervical dysplasia treated?	Laser ablation; Cryotherapy; Loop electrosurgical excision procedure (LEEP); Cervical conization

BREAST DISEASE

What is the most common benign breast condition?	Fibrocystic breast disease
What are the symptoms?	Nodularity and breast tenderness
What is a fibroadenoma?	Firm, painless, mobile masses of proliferating epithelial and fibrous tissues
Are fibroadenomas usually found in young or old women?	Young
When is surgical treatment indicated for fibroadenomas?	When the mass grows rapidly or is painful
What is an intraductal papilloma?	Epithelial tumor of the ducts

How does an intraductal papilloma present?	Spontaneous bloody, serous, or cloudy nipple discharge
What is the most common malignancy in women?	Breast cancer
What are the risk factors for developing breast cancer?	Family history (especially a first-degree relative); Decreased ovarian function (especially anovulatory menstrual cycles); Diabetes; Obesity; Nulliparity; Early menarche; Late menopause
What is the most important prognostic feature of breast cancer?	Axillary node status
What genes are associated with breast cancer?	BRCA1; BRCA2
What is the most common type of breast cancer?	Infiltrating ductal cancer (80%)
Besides infiltrating ductal cancer, what are some other types of breast cancer?	In situ and infiltrating lobular cancer; Noninfiltrating ductal cancer; Inflammatory carcinoma; Paget's disease
For which type of breast cancer is the overlying skin described as *peau d' orange* (orange peel)?	Inflammatory carcinoma
Which type of breast cancer is associated with nipple eczema and bloody discharge?	Paget's disease
What are the USPSTF recommendations for breast cancer screening?	Screening mammography every 1–2 years for women 40 years and older
What are the clinical manifestations of breast cancer?	Hard, fixed, non-tender breast; Nipple retraction; Skin erythema; Edema

OVARIAN CANCER

What is a follicular cyst?	An ovarian follicle that does not rupture during maturation, thus preventing ovulation (can result in secondary amenorrhea)
When is a follicular cyst clinically significant?	When it is large enough to cause pain or if it persists beyond one menstrual cycle

What is the management of a follicular cyst?	Repeat a pelvic examination in 6–8 weeks; OCPs (combined estrogen and progesterone) to suppress gonadotropin stimulation of the cyst; Surgery
What is a corpus luteum cyst?	A cyst that is greater than 3 cm
What are the types of glandular epithelial cell tumors?	Serous; Mucinous; Endometrioid
Which glandular epithelial cell tumors are treated with surgery?	Serous and mucinous tumors
What is the malignant potential of serous versus mucinous tumors?	30% for serous tumors and 15% for mucinous tumors
What is the most common ovarian tumor?	Benign cystic teratoma (dermoid cyst)
What are the characteristics of benign cystic teratomas?	They contain tissue from the ectoderm, mesoderm, and endoderm and can include tissue from the central nervous system, cartilage, bone, teeth, and intestinal glands
What are stromal cell tumors?	Benign tumors derived from specialized sex cord stroma (granulosa theca cell: females, Sertoli-Leydig cell: males)
What is Meigs' syndrome?	A benign ovarian fibroma (solid tumor that does not secrete sex steroids); Ascites; Right unilateral hydrothorax
What gynecological cancer has the highest mortality rate?	Ovarian cancer
What percentage of cases of ovarian cancer is associated with the BRCA1 gene?	5%
What are the types of malignant epithelial cell tumors?	Serous cystadenocarcinoma; Mucinous cystadenocarcinoma
What are the types of malignant germ cell tumors?	Dysgerminoma; Immature teratoma; Mixed germ cell tumors; Endodermal sinus tumors; Embryonal tumors
What are the types of malignant stromal cell tumors?	Granulosa cell tumor; Sertoli-Leydig cell tumors
What is the most common category of malignant ovarian neoplasms?	Malignant epithelial cell tumors (90%)
What is a Krukenberg tumor?	An ovarian tumor that is metastatic from the GI tract, breast, or endometrium

True or false: Most ovarian cancer presents at an advanced stage.	True
What is the treatment for ovarian cancer?	Primary surgical therapy (regardless of stage); Adjunctive therapy (if in advanced stage)
What is first-line chemotherapy for treatment of ovarian cancer?	Paclitaxel (Taxol); Cisplatin or carboplatin
Radiation therapy has a limited role in ovarian cancer treatment, except for in what type of malignant germ cell tumor?	Dysgerminomas

ENDOMETRIAL CANCER

What are the risk factors for endometrial cancer?	Exposure to exogenous or endogenous unopposed estrogen (i.e., without progestins); Diabetes; Hypertension (HTN)
What are examples of exogenous estrogen?	Estrogen replacement therapy; Tamoxifen
What are examples of endogenous estrogen?	Chronic anovulation secondary to polycystic ovarian syndrome (PCOS); Obesity; Estrogen-secreting tumors
What are protective factors for the development of endometrial cancer?	Oral contraceptives (progestin suppresses endometrial proliferation); Physical activity
What is the classic presentation of endometrial cancer?	Postmenopausal woman with uterine bleeding
What percentage of postmenopausal women with uterine bleeding will have endometrial cancer?	5–20%
How do perimenopausal women with endometrial cancer present?	Abnormal uterine bleeding (e.g., menometrorrhagia)
What are the diagnostic tests for endometrial cancer?	Endometrial sampling (high sensitivity); Hysteroscopy with dilation and curettage (the gold standard); Transvaginal ultrasound
True or false: Postmenopausal women with an endometrial thickness less than 5 mm have a low risk of endometrial disease.	True

MENOPAUSE

What is menopause?	The 12 months of amenorrhea after the last menstrual period
What causes menopause?	Depletion of ovarian follicles and the end of ovarian estrogen secretion
What is the average age at which menopause occurs?	51 years (90% between 45 and 55)
What is premature ovarian failure?	Menopause before the age of 40
What are common causes of premature ovarian failure?	Smoking; Chemotherapy; Hysterectomy; Low body weight; Partial deletion of the long arm of one X chromosome; Follicles resistant to follicle-stimulating hormone (FSH) and luteinizing hormone (LH); Autoantibodies against ovarian endocrine tissues
What are common clinical symptoms of perimenopause and menopause?	Changes in bleeding patterns; Menstrual migraines; Hot flashes; Sleep difficulties; Sexual dysfunction (decreased vaginal lubrication and dyspareunia); Breast tenderness; Stress and urge incontinence; Joint pain; Depression
What causes the changes in bleeding patterns?	Anovulation and progesterone deficiency
What causes the vaginal discomfort?	Decrease in estrogen causes vaginal dryness and thinning of the vaginal epithelium
What causes the stress and urge incontinence?	Atrophy of the urethral epithelium
How is menopause diagnosed?	Clinically after 12 months of amenorrhea and menopausal symptoms
True or false: A high FSH level is helpful in confirming the diagnosis of menopause.	True. But it may be suppressed after ovulation
What does HRT stand for?	Hormone replacement therapy
What are the main concerns regarding HRT according to the Women's Health Initiative?	HRT with combined estrogen-progestin increases cardiovascular risks, breast cancer, stroke, and thromboembolic disease

| Has unopposed estrogen demonstrated an increased risk of breast cancer? | No |
| What are the current recommendations for HRT? | Use at the lowest dose of estrogen for the shortest period of time possible to control menopausal symptoms |

OSTEOPOROSIS

What are main risk factors for developing osteoporosis?	Low body weight (<127 pounds); Family history; Estrogen deficiency; Low lifetime calcium intake; Current cigarette smoking; Caucasian race; High alcohol and/or caffeine intake
What is the preferred diagnostic modality for osteoporosis?	Bone mass density scan (DEXA) of the hip and spine
What is a T-score?	A representation of the patient's bone mineral density as defined by the number of standard deviations below that of a young normal adult of the same sex
What is a normal T-score?	0 to −1
What T-score defines osteopenia?	−1 to −2.5
Osteoporosis?	Less than −2.5
Severe osteoporosis?	Less than−2.5 with fragility fractures
What groups of women should get a bone mass density scan?	Older than 65 years; Postmenopausal with a new fracture; Younger than 65 years but have an additional risk factor
Men with what conditions should get a bone mass density test?	Low-trauma fractures; Radiographic osteopenia; Hypogonadism; IBD; Glucocorticoid therapy; Primary hyperparathyroidism; Loss of more than 1.5 in in height
What is the standard of treatment for osteoporosis?	Bisphosphonates; Selective estrogen receptor modulators (raloxifene); Supplemental calcium and vitamin D; Weight-bearing exercise (at least 30 minutes three times per week); Smoking cessation
How much supplemental calcium?	1000 mg per day
How much supplemental vitamin D?	400–800 IU per day

Is HRT a first-line therapy for osteoporosis?	No

UTERINE LEIOMYOMAS

What are uterine leiomyomas (fibroids)?	Benign tumors composed of uterine smooth muscle cells
What are the three types of uterine leiomyomas?	1. Submucosal 2. Intramural 3. Subserosal
Why is the incidence of fibroids higher in reproductive age women than in menopausal women?	Estrogen and progesterone increase fibroid growth
What are the risk factors for uterine leiomyomas?	Nulliparity (pregnancy promotes fibroid regression) and obesity (increased estrogen exposure); African American ethnicity
How do OCPs affect uterine leiomyomas?	Combined OCPs reduce the relative risk of fibroids
What are the three typical signs and symptoms associated with uterine leiomyomas?	1. Menorrhagia 2. Pelvic pressure and pain 3. Decreased fertility
What bimanual examination findings suggest uterine leiomyomas?	Enlarged and irregular uterus
What imaging test can be used to confirm the diagnosis of uterine leiomyomas?	Transvaginal ultrasound (95% sensitivity)
Describe the medical treatments for uterine leiomyomas.	NSAIDs for pain control; Gonadotropin releasing hormone (GnRH) agonists (e.g., leuprorelin) decrease bleeding and fibroid size; Androgens (e.g., danazol) decrease bleeding
How do danazol and GnRH agonists work?	Decrease pituitary gonadotropins
Will medicinal therapy improve fertility?	No
What are the surgical treatments for uterine leiomyomas?	Myomectomy or hysterectomy
Will a myomectomy improve fertility?	Yes
What is the name for the interventional radiology procedure for leiomyomas that injects small particles into the uterine arteries to decrease blood flow and cause regression?	Uterine artery embolization

ENDOMETRIOSIS

What is endometriosis?	Endometrial glands and stroma implanted in areas outside the endometrial cavity
At what age does endometriosis typically present?	25–35 years
Why is endometriosis rare in premenarchal and postmenopausal females?	Ectopic implants are dependent on hormones
What is the most common site for endometriosis?	Ovaries
What are the next most common sites in order of decreasing frequency?	Cul-de-sac; Broad ligament; Uterosacral ligament; Fallopian tubes; Sigmoid/appendix; Round ligaments
What are the symptoms of endometriosis?	Three Ds: **D**ysmenorrhea **D**yspareunia **D**yschezia
What usually worsens the pain of endometriosis?	Menses
Does endometriosis affect fertility?	Yes. Most patients are nulliparous
What are the signs of endometriosis on physical examination?	Tender/enlarged adnexae; A retroverted uterus; Tender nodules in the uterosacral ligaments and cul-de-sac
What is the gold standard for diagnosing endometriosis?	Direct visualization of the lesions during laparoscopy
How are endometriosis lesions described?	Raised, blue-colored mulberry spots or brown-colored powder burns
What are chocolate cysts?	Endometriomas formed when endometriosis invades the ovaries
Describe the fluid within chocolate cysts.	Thick, dark blood
What is the treatment for chocolate cysts?	Excision
Does a negative laparoscopy reliably exclude endometriosis?	Yes
Which medicines are used to treat endometriosis?	Combination oral contraceptive pills (OCPs)/progestin; Androgens (danazol); GnRH agonists

What additional class of medications can provide symptomatic relief in endometriosis?	NSAIDs
How do danazol and GnRH agonists work?	Inhibit pituitary gonadotropin secretion leading to decreased ovarian estrogen production
Are danazol and GnRH agonists as equally effective as OCPs?	Yes. But they have more side effects
What are side effects of danazol and GnRH agonists?	Hot flashes; Vaginal atrophy; Decreased bone density
When is it appropriate to refer the patient for surgery?	Failed medical management; Severe pain; Desired pregnancy
What is the conservative surgical option for patients who desire pregnancy?	Laparoscopic ablation and excision of implants and adhesions
What is the definitive surgical option?	Hysterectomy with or without salpingo-oophorectomy

VAGINITIS

What are the three most common causes of vaginitis?	1. Bacterial vaginosis (BV) 2. Vulvovaginal candidiasis 3. Trichomonas vaginalis
What is the normal vaginal pH of a woman of reproductive age?	4.0–4.5
Which common causes of vaginitis present with an elevated vaginal pH?	Bacterial vaginosis; Trichomonas
What medications or practices can alter the normal vaginal pH?	Antibiotics; OCPs; Sexual activity; Douching
How does normal physiologic vaginal discharge in a reproductive age woman appear?	White; Thick; Odorless; Less than 4 mL per 24 hours
What are some nonpathogenic causes of an increased amount of vaginal discharge?	Pregnancy; OCP use; Ovulation
What are the most important tests to diagnose vaginitis?	Vaginal pH and microscopy (saline wet mount and 10% KOH preps)
What bacteria are normally found in the vagina of a reproductive age woman?	*Lactobacilli* (predominant); *Gardnerella vaginalis; Staphylococcus epidermidis; Escherichia coli; Candida albicans;* group B *streptococcus*
Why does the vaginal pH increase in BV?	*Lactobacilli,* which produce lactic acid, are decreased in BV

Which type of cells will you see on the saline (wet mount) prep with BV?

"Clue cells" (vaginal squamous epithelial cells covered with bacteria)

Which type of smell will you notice with the KOH prep in BV?

An amine smell, known as the "whiff test"

What are Amstel's criteria for diagnosing BV?

Abnormal gray discharge (often fishy smelling); Vaginal pH >4.5; Positive amine "whiff test"; >20% clue cells[*]

How do you treat BV?

Metronidazole (500 mg, PO bid × 7 days) or clindamycin, both of which are safe in pregnancy

How does vulvovaginal candidiasis present?

Vulvar itching; Burning; Dyspareunia; Dysuria; Whitish thick "cottage cheese" discharge

What do you see on microscopy in candidiasis (albicans-species)?

Fungal blastospores and pseudohyphae, seen with both saline and KOH mounts

Why is KOH mount preferred over a saline mount?

KOH destroys other cellular elements

How do you treat uncomplicated candidiasis?

Topical or oral azoles, commonly oral fluconazole; Advise patient to avoid nylon or tight-fitting clothing

How do you treat severe candidiasis?

Give a second dose of oral fluconazole three days after first dose

How do you treat recurrent candidiasis?

Daily oral fluconazole for 7–14 days, then weekly for six months

What is the best method for treating candidiasis in pregnancy?

Topical azole therapy for seven days

How does trichomonas appear under microscopy?

Motile, flagellated trichomonads on saline prep if checked <20 minutes after specimen obtained

How is trichomonas spread?

Sexual contact

How do you treat trichomonas?

Metronidazole (2 g PO × 1); Treat the sexual partner also

What should patients avoid when taking metronidazole to avoid disulfiram reaction?

Alcohol

Trichomonas can cause what complications of pregnancy?

Preterm delivery; Premature rupture of membranes; Low birth weight

[*]Three out of four criteria must be present to diagnose BV

CERVICITIS/PELVIC INFLAMMATORY DISEASE, AND SEXUALLY TRANSMITTED INFECTIONS

How can you differentiate between urethritis from sexually transmitted infections (STIs) versus urinary tract infections (UTIs)?

STI: Nitrite negative; Culture negative

UTI: Nitrite may be elevated; + Blood; + Culture

Both: Pyuria; Positive leukocyte esterase

Which STI is the most prevalent in the United States?

Chlamydia

For which groups of women does the Centers for Disease Control and Prevention (CDC) recommend annual chlamydial screening?

All sexually active women aged 25 years or younger; Sexually active women older than 25 with risk factors (new sexual partner, more than one sexual partner in the past three months, or inconsistent use of barrier contraceptives)

If a patient has chlamydia, what other STI should you empirically treat for?

Gonorrhea

How is chlamydia cervicitis treated?

Azithromycin (1 g PO × 1); Doxycycline (100 mg PO bid × 7 days)

How is gonorrhea cervicitis treated?

Ceftriaxone (125 mg IM × 1); Ciprofloxacin (500 mg PO × 1)

What are some symptoms of cervicitis?

Vaginal discharge; Dysuria; Dyspareunia; Minor vaginal bleeding

What are some infectious causes of cervicitis?

Gonorrhea and chlamydia; Trichomonas; Herpes; *Mycoplasma genitalium*

How does cervicitis appear on speculum examination?

Cervical or urethral discharge; Erythema; Friable cervix

With which normal finding of the cervix must cervicitis not be confused?

Ectropion

What is ectropion?

Eversion of columnar cervical epithelium over the external os, often caused by oral contraceptives and found in adolescents

What is the definition of PID?

Acute, usually polymicrobic, infection/inflammation of the upper genital tract in women, involving any or all of the uterus, oviducts, ovaries, and pelvic peritoneum

How does cervicitis lead to PID?	By ascending infection of microorganisms
What are the most common organisms found to cause PID?	*Neisseria gonorrhoeae; Chlamydia trachomatis; Mycoplasma genitalium;* Anaerobic and facultative organisms (*Prevotella, E. coli, Haemophilus influenzae,* group B *streptococcus*)
How does PID typically present?	Lower abdominal pain (90%); Mucopurulent cervical discharge (75%); Fever (50%); Rebound tenderness; Urethritis; Proctitis; Chills; Abnormal uterine bleeding
What are the three major determinants that must be present to diagnose PID?	1. Lower abdominal pain and tenderness 2. Cervical motion tenderness 3. Adnexal tenderness (may be unilateral)
What are some of the minor determinants that lead to a diagnosis of PID?	Fever >101°F; Vaginal discharge; Documented STI; Systemic signs; Dyspareunia
What laboratory tests should you perform if you suspect PID in a patient?	Pregnancy test; Microscopy of discharge; CBC; Gonorrhea (GC)/Chlamydia tests; Urinalysis
What study should you perform if the patient appears acutely ill with a pelvic mass?	Pelvic ultrasound to rule out a tubo-ovarian abscess (TOA)
What are the sequelae of untreated PID?	Ectopic pregnancy; Infertility; Chronic pelvic pain; Recurrent salpingitis
Which patients should you hospitalize for treatment of PID?	Pregnant; Adolescent; Poorly compliant; Immunodeficient; Nausea/vomiting/high fever; TOA; Upper peritoneal signs; Inadequate response to outpatient therapy after 48 hours; Uncertain diagnosis
What are some recommended outpatient regimens for treatment of PID?	Appropriate antibiotics for two weeks; Treat the partner also

CONTRACEPTION

How does progesterone work as a contraceptive?	Suppresses LH to prevent ovulation; Produces an atrophied endometrium to prevent ovum implantation;

	Thickens the cervical mucus to prevent sperm transport; Inhibits peristalsis of fallopian tubes
How does estrogen work as a contraceptive?	Suppresses FSH to prevent emergence of a dominant follicle; Provides stability to the endometrium to prevent breakthrough bleeding; Potentiates the action of progesterone
How many weeks postpartum should a woman wait before resuming intercourse?	Six weeks
Which hormone should be avoided during exclusive breastfeeding because it decreases milk production?	Estrogen
What are the best birth control options for a breastfeeding woman?	Barrier methods; Progesterone-only pill (POP); Depo-medroxyprogesterone (DMPA) injection; Intrauterine device (IUD)
In a nonlactating woman, how early postpartum can you start an estrogen-containing contraceptive without increased risk of thrombosis?	Three weeks postpartum
How long can lactational amenorrhea work as an effective birth control method?	Up to six months, *only* if the woman is breast-feeding exclusively both day and night and she is still amenorrheic (not 100% effective)
At what time during her menstrual cycles should you instruct a woman to begin a pack of OCPs (or other hormonal contraceptive)?	On the first day of menses or the first Sunday after menses
Is this a hard and fast rule?	No. They can start it any time, but should use a backup method for one week to one month if they do not start it then
Do women have to take "breaks" from being on hormonal birth control?	No. Women who are healthy and do not smoke can use hormonal birth control continuously from menarche until menopause if they desire
Can women who prefer not to have their menses every month skip the one-week break and start their next pill pack/patch/ring after three-week of use?	Yes
In terms of birth control, what does "typical use" rate mean?	The rate takes people's actual birth control habits (not always using birth control correctly) into account

What percentage of sexually active women, using the following methods of birth control, will experience an unintended pregnancy in one year?[*]

No birth control	85%
Periodic abstinence only (natural family planning)	25%
Male condoms only	15%
OCPs, the Ortho Evra patch, or the NuvaRing	8%
Depot-medroxyprogesterone acetate (DMPA) injections	3%
IUD	Less than 1% (0.8% with ParaGard, 0.1% with Mirena)

Which form of sterilization is more effective, male or female?
Male, although the failure rate is low for both (male—0.15%, female—0.5%)

In which type of women are cervical caps most effective?
Nulliparous women

Which lubricants are safe to use with latex condoms?
Water-based or silicone gels

Which are not safe to use and why?
Oils, petroleum jelly, and antibiotic vaginal creams may cause the condom to break

Condoms are effective at preventing or reducing the transmission of which sexually transmitted infections?
HIV; Gonorrhea; Chlamydia; Trichomonas; Syphilis; Herpes; Chancroid; HPV

Which birth control method has been shown to increase transmission of HIV?
Nonoxynol-9 spermicide by causing small tears in the vaginal epithelium

Which birth control methods have both estrogen and progesterone components?
Combined oral contraceptives (COCs); Ortho Evra patch; NuvaRing

Which birth control methods contain progesterone, but no estrogen?
Progesterone-only pills (Micronor); DMPA injection; Mirena IUD

Which cancers have a proven associated decreased risk with COC use?
Endometrial cancers; Ovarian cancers; Colorectal cancers

What other medical benefits do COCs offer?
Reduced risk of ectopic pregnancy and PID; Treatment for acne, hirsutism, and androgen excess; Reduced vasomotor symptoms in

[*]These statistics are based on "typical use" rates

perimenopausal women; Increased bone mineral density; Decreased risk of hemorrhagic corpus luteum cysts; Reduction in benign breast disease

What risks are associated with COCs?

Increased risk of cervical adenocarcinoma (rare) and hepatic adenoma; Increased risk of venous thromboembolism; Increased risk of myocardial infarction (MI) and stroke in smokers over 35 years old or patients with a history of HTN, diabetes, hyperlipidemia, obesity; Severe migraines; Reversible HTN; Cholelithiasis

What side effects might COC users experience?

Increased headaches; Nausea; Vomiting; Breast tenderness/pain; Varicosities; Average weight gain is no more than in placebo users

How often do the Ortho Evra patch and NuvaRing have to be changed?

Ortho Evra Patch: once a week

NuvaRing: once a month

How often do DMPA injections need to be given for effective contraception?

Every three months

How does DMPA affect menstruation?

Irregular menstruation during first several months and then possible amenorrhea thereafter

What are some possible side effects of DMPA use?

Weight gain; Acne; Hirsutism; Hair loss; Mood changes; Decreased bone mineral density

How does the ParaGard Copper T IUD work?

Copper ions inhibit sperm motility and a sterile inflammatory reaction created in the endometrium kills the sperm

For how long after insertion is the ParaGard Copper T IUD effective?

12 years (approved for 10 years)

How does the Mirena IUD work?

Contains progesterone which thickens cervical mucus, alters endometrium, changes uterotubal fluid to impair sperm migration, and sometimes causes anovulation

For how long after insertion is the Mirena IUD effective?

At least five years

Who should use the IUDs?

Recommended for women in stable mutually monogamous relationships

	(low STI risk) who want reversible long-term contraception
What side effects may be experienced with IUDs?	Increased dysmenorrhea and blood loss (during first few months and more often with ParaGard); Amenorrhea (after one year with Mirena)
Do ParaGard or Mirena increase the risk for PID?	Only during the first 20 days after insertion
Approximately what percentage of pregnancies in the United States are unintended?	About 50%
As of 2000, what percentage of unintended pregnancies ended in an elective abortion?	About 50%, or 25% of all pregnancies
What options are available for a woman who has just discovered she has an unintended pregnancy?	Continuation of pregnancy; Adoption; Elective abortion (some states require parental notification and/or consent for teens)
What is emergency contraception?	High-dose hormones given to prevent pregnancy after a contraceptive fails or after unprotected sex
What are the options for emergency contraception?	0.75 mg levonorgestrel within 72 hours of having sex, then again 12 hours later (Plan B); 0.5 mg levonorgestrel and 100 µg of ethinyl estradiol within 120 hours of having sex, then again 12 hours later
What is the name of the only Food and Drug Administration (FDA)-approved emergency contraception pill being sold in the United States today?	Plan B
How does Plan B work?	Stops ovulation; May prevent fertilization; May prevent implantation
Who may purchase Plan B over-the-counter?	Men and women over the age of 18 years (women under 17 need a prescription)

INFERTILITY

| What is infertility? | Failure to conceive after one year of unprotected sex |

What percentage of couples experience infertility?	15%
What is the monthly probability of pregnancy among fertile couples?	20%
What is the cumulative probability of pregnancy among fertile couples after 12 months?	93%
What are common causes of a female etiology for infertility?	Anovulation or oligoovulation; Aging oocytes; Tubal interruption such as PID, pelvic adhesions, or endometriosis; Uterine abnormalities such as submucosal fibroid, septate uterus, endometrial polyp, or synechiae
What are the options for diagnosing the cause of infertility?	See Table 16.1
How can you induce ovulation in an anovulatory patient?	Clomiphene citrate and gonadotropins
What is clomiphene citrate?	A weak estrogen that works as an anti-estrogen
How does it work?	Blocks estrogen receptors and causes negative feedback on the hypothalamic- pituitary-ovarian axis and an increase in FSH secretion

Table 16.1 Infertility Diagnostic Tests

	Cause of infertility	Test
Male	Azoospermia	Semen analysis (semen volume, sperm concentration, motility, and morphology)
Female	Anovulation	Midluteal serum progesterone level
		Urine LH surge detection
		Basal body temperature curve ($\uparrow$ progesterone $\rightarrow$ $\uparrow$ 0.5–1°F)
	Uterine abnormality	Hysterosalpingography
		Hysteroscopy
		Ultrasound (for visualization of fibroids)
	Tubal obstruction	Hysterosalpingography
		Laparoscopy

PREGNANCY

How soon after conception can a urine pregnancy test be positive?	7–10 days
Which hormone is used in pregnancy test to determine if a woman is pregnant?	Beta-human chorionic gonadotrophin (β-hCG)
Urine and pregnancy tests can detect pregnancy at what level of β-hCG?	Urine: 25 mIU/mL Serum: 5 mIU/mL
How often does β-hCG double during normal pregnancy?	1.5 days before 5 weeks; 2 days between 5 weeks and 7 weeks
What is the most accurate technique for determining gestational age?	Measurement of the crown-rump length at 7–14 weeks by ultrasound
What is the β-hCG threshold at which transvaginal ultrasound should reveal an intrauterine pregnancy?	1500–2000 mIU/mL
When the β-hCG is above this threshold and there is no pregnancy seen on ultrasound, the possibility of what should be considered?	Ectopic pregnancy
When can fetal heart tones be initially heard using Doppler?	9–12 weeks
What initial prenatal lab tests does ACOG recommend?	Blood type/Rh and antibody screen (ABO/Rh); Hemoglobin and hematocrit; Pap smear; Rubella titer; Syphilis screen; Urine analysis and culture; hepatitis B surface antigen; HIV; Chlamydia; Gonorrhea
What is the recommended dosage of folic acid during the early prenatal period?	400 μg
What is the recommended average weight gain for women with the following body mass index (BMI)?	
BMI <19.8	28–40 lb
BMI 19.8–26.0	25–35 lb (an average of 300 kcal/day)
BMI > 26.0	15–25 lb
What are the recommended second and third trimester prenatal labs?	"Triple screen" = alpha fetoprotein (AFP), estriol, free β-hCG (16–20-weeks gestation); one-hour glucose challenge (24–28 weeks gestation); Group B *streptococcus* culture (33–37-weeks gestation)

What drug is used to prevent maternal sensitization to Rh D antigens?

RhoGAM

> **Is RhoGAM given to mothers who are Rh negative or positive?**

Negative

> **When is RhoGAM given?**

Once at 28–30 weeks gestation, then again soon after delivery if the baby is Rh positive (also given with trauma, bleeding, and spontaneous abortion)

What is preeclampsia?

New onset of HTN and proteinuria after 20-weeks gestation

How do you diagnose preeclampsia?

SBP >140 mm Hg OR DBP >90 mm Hg *and* 24-hour urine protein is 0.3 g or greater

What are common risk factors for preeclampsia?

Nulliparity; Preeclampsia in previous pregnancy; Teenager or age >35 years; African American or Hispanic; Positive family history; Chronic HTN; Chronic renal disease; Antiphospholipid antibody; Diabetes mellitus; Vascular or connective tissue disease; Multiple gestations; High BMI

What are other end-organ manifestations of preeclampsia?

Increased platelet turnover; Glomerular and hepatic injury from vasospasm; Headache; Blurred vision; Scotoma

What is HELLP syndrome?

A severe form of preeclampsia when a patient develops **h**emolysis, **e**levated **l**iver enzymes, and **l**ow **p**latelets

What is eclampsia?

The development of seizures in a preeclamptic patient

What is the definitive treatment for preeclampsia or eclampsia?

Delivery of the fetus

What medication is used to prevent seizures in preeclampsia?

Magnesium sulfate

What is the puerperium?

The 6–8-week period postpartum when the body gradually returns to its nonpregnant state

What is lochia?

Vaginal discharge immediately after delivery from blood clots expelled from the uterus and decidua that gradually sloughs off

When does ovulation postpartum resume in non–breast-feeding women?

Ten weeks on an average

When does ovulation postpartum resume in breast-feeding women?

Depends on how long she nurses and can sometimes be up to six months

What is the mean weight loss immediately after delivery?

13 lb from delivery of the fetus, placenta, and amniotic fluid

How long does it take for the uterus to return to its nonpregnant size?

6–8 weeks

In the United States, what are the contraindications to breast-feeding?

Mother has HIV or HTLV-1 (human T-cell lymphotropic virus), abused drugs, or is taking antineoplastic or antimetabolic drugs; Infant has galactosemia

What is breast engorgement?

Swelling of the breast from edema and/or accumulated milk

What are common infections during the postpartum period?

Endometritis; UTI; Mastitis; Wound infection; Pelvic thrombophlebitis

CHAPTER 17

Pediatrics

NEWBORNS AND INFANTS

What is a term infant?	A baby born between 37-weeks- and 42-weeks gestation
Premature	Less than 37 weeks
Post-term	More than 42 weeks
What is an APGAR score?	A measure of the general well-being of a newborn
When are APGAR scores measured?	At one and five minutes after birth
When should APGAR scores be repeated if the initial scores are less than 7?	At 10, 15, and 20 minutes after birth
What are the five APGAR categories?	1. Heart rate 2. Respiratory effort 3. Muscle tone 4. Reflex irritability 5. Color
What is the maximum number of points on the APGAR score?	There are up to 2 points in each category for a maximum of 10 points
True or false: The one-minute APGAR determines what kind of resuscitation the newborn needs.	False. Some babies need resuscitation much sooner
How many vessels does a normal umbilical cord have?	Three (two arteries and one vein)
What is the typical weight of a healthy newborn?	2.5–4 kg
Length	46–54 cm
FOC (head circumference)	32–38 cm
What is the definition of low birth weight (LBW)?	Less than 2500 g at birth
What are the causes of LBW?	Intrauterine growth restriction (IUGR); Prematurity; Normal variant

What is the predominant cause of LBW in the United States?	Prematurity
What are the factors associated with IUGR (estimated fetal weight < 10th percentile)?	Genetic abnormalities; Multiple gestation; Fetal insulin deficiency; Placental insufficiency; Maternal disease (e.g., HTN, sickle cell disease); Drug use
What is large for gestational age (LGA)?	Larger than 90th percentile for gestational age
What is the weight of a term LGA baby?	More than 4000 g
What is the most common cause of LGA babies?	Maternal diabetes
Normal newborns may lose up to what percentage of their weight in the first week of life?	Up to 10%
By how many weeks of age should a healthy baby be back to birth weight?	Two weeks
In the first couple of months, about how much weight should a baby gain per day?	1 oz (or 28 g)
True or false: A normal baby's respiratory rate and heart rate are slower than those of a normal adult.	False
True or false: A normal baby's blood pressure is lower than that of a normal adult.	True
True or false: Doing a good initial heart examination rules out heart abnormalities.	False
Why?	Some abnormalities may not be evident initially (example: high pulmonary artery (PA) pressures on day one may diminish L → R shunting, so murmur of a ventricular septal defect (VSD) is non-appreciable)
When does the anterior fontanelle close?	During second year of life
Posterior fontanelle	First few months of life
What is head "molding" in a newborn?	Irregularly shaped head with palpable ridges
What causes it?	Pressure in the birth canal during labor and delivery
How long does it normally last?	It should disappear within a week
What is caput succedaneum?	Diffuse soft tissue edema of the scalp

What causes it?	Pressure on presenting part of scalp during delivery
Does it require treatment?	No. It resolves on its own in a few days
What is cephalohematoma?	Subperiosteal hemorrhage
What usually causes it?	Small tearing of vessels during delivery
What are worrisome causes?	Skull fracture; Coagulopathy; Intracerebral hemorrhage
What kind of treatment does an uncomplicated cephalohematoma require?	Usually none (resolves on its own), but may need treatment for hyperbilirubinemia from blood reabsorption
Which crosses suture lines, cephalohematoma or caput succedaneum?	Caput succedaneum
What does an absent red reflex indicate?	Something is inhibiting light from getting to the retina (e.g., cataract, tumor)
Intermittent strabismus is normal up until what age?	Three months
What is the most common birth defect?	Hearing loss
What procedures are available to screen infants for hearing loss?	Measurement of otoacoustic emissions (OAEs) and/or auditory brain response (ABR)
Why is it so important to test for hearing loss?	Hearing loss can significantly delay a child's development, especially language acquisition
Small, low-set, or floppy ears may be a sign of what other abnormalities?	Chromosomal abnormality; Renal abnormality
A common benign newborn rash consisting of small white papules on a blotchy erythematous base is called what?	Erythema toxicum
What is the required treatment?	None (disappears on its own)
How long does it typically take an umbilical cord stump to fall off?	1–3 weeks
A female baby has swollen nipples and white vaginal discharge with a tinge of blood. Is this normal?	Yes
What is the cause?	Baby's exposure to maternal hormones

What is the American Academy of Pediatrics' stance on routine circumcision?	Not medically necessary
The Ortolani and Barlow maneuvers test for what abnormality?	Developmental hip dysplasia
What are some late diagnostic signs of developmental hip dysplasia?	Asymmetry of the following: thigh folds, hip abduction, and/or knee height
Lumbosacral dimples or hair tufts are concerning for what type of abnormality?	Underlying vertebral/spinal cord abnormality (e.g., neural tube defect)
Stroking the sole of the foot normally causes an infant's toes to go up or down?	Up
Stroking a newborn's cheek causes him to turn his head to the same side and make sucking motions with his mouth. What is this called?	Rooting reflex
When does the Moro reflex (startle reflex) normally disappear?	3–4 months
True or false: Every U.S. state has a newborn screening program for metabolic and other inherited disorders.	True
Most state newborn screens include testing for what disorders?	Hypothyroidism; Phenylketonuria; Galactosemia; Sickle cell disease
What is the most common chromosomal abnormality?	Down syndrome (Trisomy 21)
What are the most frequent causes of death in infants (<12 months old)?	Sudden infant death syndrome (SIDS); Perinatal conditions (e.g., complications of prematurity); Congenital abnormalities; Chromosomal abnormalities
About how many hours does a newborn sleep per 24 hours?	16–20

INFANT FEEDING

Ideally, when should breast-feeding begin?	If possible, right after birth
What are the intrinsic benefits of breast milk compared to infant formula?	Composed of macro- and micronutrients specific and ideal for human babies, breast milk provides

*Tip: When you begin examining a newborn and s/he is not crying, take advantage of the opportunity to auscultate the heart and lungs and check for a red reflex

maternal antibodies (decreasing infections), is less expensive, and more environment friendly

What additional benefits may be conferred to a breast-fed baby?

Decreased incidence of SIDS, lymphoma, malignancies, obesity, diabetes, and allergies/eczema; Increased IQ scores

What additional benefits of breast-feeding may be conferred to mothers?

Contracts uterus; Helps in returning to pre-pregnancy weight; Delay of menses; "Feel-good" hormone release (oxytocin); Decreased incidence of breast cancer, ovarian cancer, and osteoporosis later in life

How often should a breast-fed infant feed?

8–12 times every 24 hours until four months of age

How long should each feeding last?

10–15 minutes on each breast

What is the current recommendation regarding breast-feeding in the developed world if the mother is HIV+?

Baby should be formula-fed because of risk for infection via breast milk

How can we promote breast-feeding?

Education pre- and post-delivery about the benefits of breast-feeding, reinforcement, and early lactation training (proper latch-on techniques)

The American Academy of Pediatrics recommends breast-feeding for how long?

12 months

What can be used as a supplement or alternative to breast milk?

Formula (cow-milk or soy-milk based)

The standard formula for a term infant has how many kilocalories per ounce?

20 kcal/oz

How many ounces should a formula-fed baby feed in the first few months of life?

On *average*, 2–3 oz every 3–4 hours by two weeks of age, progressively increasing to 5–6 oz every 3–4 hours at six months of age

How do you know if a baby is eating enough?

Plotting weight; Length; FOC on a development curve

How early may a baby be introduced to solid foods?

Four months

For how long may a baby's nutritional needs be met by formula or breast milk alone?

Six months

What are the signs that a baby is ready to eat solid foods? Head control; Loss of extrusion reflex; Still hungry after consuming 32 oz of formula or nursing ten times per day

What types of food are appropriate for an infant beginning to eat solids? Food that is soft and easy to digest (rice cereal with iron)

How should these foods be introduced? Slowly and no more than one new food every three days

Do all babies spit up? Generally all babies will spit up at some time during feeds

Why? Babies have low esophageal sphincter tone; Caretakers overfeed or inadequately burp them

When is reflux worrisome? Spitting up happens all of the time; Weight gain is inadequate; The reflux causes the baby to cry incessantly, cough, or wheeze

What should be the primary source of nutrition for a baby up to one year of age? Breast milk or formula (solids are only a supplement)

What foods should be avoided in babies less than 12 months old? Potent allergens such as egg whites, cow milk, honey, nut butters, citrus fruit, and seafood (especially shellfish)

Which of these can cause infant botulism poisoning? Honey

What types of food should be avoided in children less than three years old? Anything that may cause the toddler to choke (peanuts, whole grapes, raw vegetables that snap into hard chunks, etc.)

What teeth are usually the first to erupt? Mandibular central incisors

When (on average)? 6–8 months

GROWTH AND DEVELOPMENT

What parameters should you plot on a growth chart at each well-child visit? Weight and length/height until adulthood and FOC the first two years

Why is it important to plot these values over time? The overall pattern of growth (i.e., *trajectory* of the curve) is more important than the raw values

What is the most common cause of obesity in children? Overeating and inactivity

Increased incidence of obesity has led to an increased incidence of what other diseases among children?	DM II; HTN; Hyperlipidemia
A BMI at what percentile defines "overweight?"	85th–95th (age-specific)
"Obese"	Greater than 95th (age-specific)
What is "failure to thrive (FTT)?"	Inappropriately low weight (< 3rd–5th percentile for the patient's age); Growth curve that crosses two major percentiles; Loss of weight
What accounts for 60–80% of FTT?	Nonorganic and psychosocial causes (e.g., poverty, neglect, mother with postpartum depression)
What are the organic causes of FTT?	Any medical condition that can cause inadequate caloric intake, absorption, or utilization (e.g., gastroesophageal reflux disease [GERD], cystic fibrosis, food allergies, metabolic storage diseases); Increased metabolic need (e.g., congenital heart disease, chronic infection)
What is the treatment of FTT?	Frequent meals; Increasing high-calorie solid food intake with additional supplementation if necessary; Treatment of underlying medical condition
What are the benefits of assessing a child's physical, social, and cognitive development?	Delays are relatively easy to detect and give important information about a child's health
What is the Denver Developmental Screening Test?	A brief developmental assessment tool to screen 0–6-year-olds
When assessing the development of a baby born prematurely, up until what age do you adjust his/her chronological age?	Two years
A nine-month-old baby who was born three months prematurely should be able to perform at what developmental level?	A six-month old
Approximately, at what age should a/n infant/child have the following gross motor skills?	
While prone, lift head to 90°	3–4 months
Roll front to back	Four months

Sit up with back unsupported	Six months
Crawl, cruise, and pull to a stand	Nine months
Take first steps	12 months
Walk up the stairs supported by wall or railing	18 months
Run well	Two years
Ride a tricycle	Three years

Approximately, at what age should an infant/child have the following fine motor skills?

Purposefully grasp an object	4–5 months
Pincer grasp	Nine months
Copy a line	Two years
Copy a circle	Three years
Copy a square	Four years

Approximately, at what age should a/n infant/child have the following language skills?

Coo	2–3 months
Babble	Six months
Say one or two distinct words	9–12 months
Follow one-step commands	12–15 months
Use 2–3-word phrases	Two years
Speak half intelligibly to a stranger	Two years
Speak three-fourths intelligibly to a stranger	Three years
Speak 100% intelligibly	Four years
Name four colors and four body parts	Four years

Approximately, at what age should a/n infant/child have the following social cognition skills?

Social smile	Two months
Laugh and squeal	Four months
Wave "bye-bye"	Ten months
Play alongside—but not with—other children (parallel play)	Two years

Play with a group of other children	Three years
On *average*, at what age do most babies begin to sleep 5–6 hours at a time?	Six months
When does stranger and separation anxiety usually begin?	7–9 months
When should toilet training *begin* in a child?	Every child is different, but usually between 18–30 months
Bed-wetting is normal up to what age?	Four years in girls and five years in boys

ADOLESCENTS

What do the Tanner Stages measure?	Sexual maturity
How many Tanner Stages are there?	Five
What is Tanner Stage 1?	Preadolescent
What is Tanner Stage 5?	Adult
What is the first visible sign of puberty in girls?	Appearance of breast buds, usually between 8–13 years
What physical changes follow?	Skeletal growth; Pubic and axillary hair; Menarche
When is menarche in relation to breast bud appearance?	About 2–2$\frac{1}{2}$ years later
What is the classic triad of McCune-Albright syndrome?	1. Polyostotic fibrous dysplasia 2. Café-au-lait spots 3. Precocious puberty
What is delayed sexual development in girls?	No breast development by the age of 14
What is primary amenorrhea?	No menarche by 16 years
What is the first visible sign of puberty in boys?	Testicular enlargement
What physical changes follow?	Pubic hair; Enlargement of penis; Spermarche; Skeletal and muscle growth
What is delayed sexual development in boys?	No testicular enlargement by 16 years
What is the most common cause of delayed puberty?	Constitutional delay (a normal variant)
What labs do you use to evaluate delayed puberty if you suspect it is due to	Follicle-stimulating hormone (FSH); Luteinizing hormone (LH); Estradiol

a disorder of the hypothalamic-pituitary-gonadal axis?	(in girls) or testosterone (in boys)
What tests do you order if these are abnormal?	GnRH stimulation test and consider MRI to rule out cranial lesions
What is the most common chromosomal cause of delayed puberty in girls?	Turner's syndrome (XO)—patients have gonadal dysgenesis
What physical examination findings may be seen in Turner's syndrome?	Short stature; Inner canthal folds with ptosis; Short-webbed neck; Widely-spaced nipples; Shield-like chest; Lymphedema of the hands and feet
What are the three common cardiac defects associated with Turner's syndrome?	1. Coarctation of the aorta 2. Bicuspid aortic valve 3. Aortic stenosis
What is the most common chromosomal cause of delayed puberty in boys?	Klinefelter's syndrome (XXY)
What physical examination findings are seen in Klinefelter's syndrome?	Tall stature with a height: arm span ratio of >1; Small testes/penis; Gynecomastia
What are the characteristics of Kallmann syndrome?	Hypogonadotropic hypogonadism; Anosmia or hyposmia; Delayed puberty; Small penis in boys; Lack of breast development in girls
When evaluating an adolescent, what does the acronym "HEADSS" stand for?	Home, Education and Employment, Activity, Drugs, Sexuality, and Suicide and Depression
What is the significance of the "HEADSS" mnemonic?	Builds a rapport; Obtains information about risk exposure; Guides preventive measures, including education on sensitive topics
What are the top three causes of death among adolescents?	1. Unintentional injury/trauma 2. Homicide 3. Suicide

SAFETY AND PREVENTION

What general signs and symptoms of illness in a baby should parents learn to recognize?	Fever; Poor feeding; Decreased urine output; Diarrhea; Vomiting; Inconsolable crying
What is the most common cause of death in children?	Unintentional injury

What bath safety tips should be given to all caregivers?	Set water heaters at lower than 120°F to prevent scalding burns and *never* leave children unattended
Why should infants be placed to sleep on their backs?	To help reduce the risk of sudden infant death syndrome (SIDS)
How long should a baby's car seat face backward?	Until the child is at least one year old *and* weighs at least 20 lb
True or false: It is OK if caregivers smoke as long as it is only outdoors.	False. Smoking outdoors does not adequately eliminate second-hand smoking exposure
Exposure to passive smoking has been linked to an increased incidence of what problems in infants and children?	Growth retardation; Respiratory and ear infections; Asthma; SIDS
True or false: You should not report child abuse unless you have proof.	False. It is *mandatory* to report abuse, even if it is only a suspicion of abuse
Overexposure to lead can have what significant health effects on children?	Low levels: Behavior and cognitive problems (e.g., learning disabilities) High levels: Anemia; Colic; Nephropathy; Encephalopathy; Even death
When should an initial lead screening be done?	At 12 months of age in low-risk children and earlier (about six months) in high-risk children
What factors can place a child at high-risk for lead exposure?	Living in or regularly visiting a house built before 1950; Living in or regularly visiting a house built before 1978 that has had recent renovation (last six months); Living near an industry that releases lead (such as a battery plant)
What is a normal lead level (in µg/dL)?	No measurable level of lead is normal

CARDIOLOGY

What causes the sound of a murmur?	Turbulent blood flow
Name five innocent murmurs of childhood.	1. Still's 2. Peripheral pulmonic stenosis (PPS) 3. Carotid innominate bruit 4. Venous hum 5. Pulmonary outflow murmur
What does Still's murmur sound like?	Musical; Twangy; Like a rubber band loudest at the apex

Where does the PPS radiate?	It is an ejection murmur that radiates to the axilla and backs
When does PPS disappear?	6–12 months
What is a PDA?	Patent ductus arteriosus (connection remains between the aorta and pulmonary artery)
What does the murmur sound like?	A continuous machine-like murmur
When does the ductus usually close?	Early in the neonatal period
What does sweating with feeds suggest?	The presence of a congenital heart defect
In order, what are the most common congenital cardiac defects?	Ventral septal defect (VSD); Pulmonary stenosis; Atrial septal defect (ASD); Coarctation of the aorta
Why might the murmur of VSD not be appreciable on the first day of life?	High PA pressures on day one may diminish L→R shunting
What physical examination findings are important in helping rule out coarctation of the aorta?	Good palpable femoral pulses; Equal upper and lower extremity blood pressure; Well-perfused lower extremities
What are the congenitally acquired *cyanotic* heart abnormalities?	Truncus arteriosus; Transposition of the great vessels; Tricuspid atresia; Tetralogy of Fallot; Total anomalous pulmonary venous return
Acyanotic	VSD; ASD; Patent ductus arteriosus (PDA)
What is the most common cause of sudden cardiac death in young athletes?	Hypertrophic cardiomyopathy

JAUNDICE AND HYPERBILIRUBINEMIA

What is jaundice?	Yellowed skin and sclera secondary to increased levels of bilirubin
Where on the body can you first note jaundice and how does it then progress?	It starts in the gums and sclera, then progresses cephalocaudally. As bilirubin decreases, the jaundice recedes in the opposite direction
Jaundice appears as a physical sign when bilirubin levels reach what concentration?	5 mg/dL
What percent of term newborn infants have jaundice sometime during the first week of life?	60%

Premature newborns	80%
Why is jaundice appearing within the first day of life so worrisome?	It is *always* pathologic
What is the differential diagnosis of jaundice on the first day of life?	Erythroblastosis fetalis; Concealed hemorrhage; Sepsis; Intrauterine infection (e.g., toxoplasmosis, rubella, cytomegalovirus [CMV], syphilis)
Describe physiologic jaundice of the newborn.	Breakdown of fetal RBCs + immature liver's inability to conjugate hemoglobin efficiently = jaundice secondary to rise in bilirubin (<5 mg/dL per day)
When does is peak?	Second to fourth day of life
When does it resolve?	Between fifth day and seventh day
What clues might suggest that a newborn's jaundice is *not* physiologic?	Appears in the first 24–36 hours of life; Bilirubin rises at >5 mg/dL per day, total is >12 mg/dL; Jaundice lasts more than 10–14 days; Conjugated bilirubin level is >2 mg/dL at any time
What is the fatal complication of hyperbilirubinemia?	Kernicterus
What is kernicterus?	Brain damage from unbound unconjugated bilirubin crossing the blood brain barrier. It results in apoptosis and necrosis
Which is neurotoxic, conjugated or unconjugated bilirubin?	Unconjugated
What concentration of bilirubin is considered "hyperbilirubinemia"?	12 mg/dL
At what level of total unconjugated bilirubin do you initiate treatment?	Depends on the newborn's age and risk factors, though generally between 11 mg/dL and 20 mg/dL
How is it most commonly treated?	Phototherapy
How does phototherapy work?	"Bili lights" are at a wavelength that converts bilirubin into a photoisomer that the body has an easier time excreting
Describe breast-feeding failure jaundice versus breast milk jaundice.	
Breast-feeding failure jaundice	An exaggeration of physiologic jaundice; Peaks within the first few

days of life; Is due to poor initial milk production and increased enterohepatic circulation; Treated by increasing breast milk feedings

Breast milk jaundice

It starts at 3–5 days, peaks at 2 weeks, and may be due to intrinsic factors in breast milk, which increase enterohepatic circulation

GASTROENTEROLOGY

When do umbilical hernias usually close?

Often in the first year, but it can take 2–3 years

When is surgical intervention of an umbilical hernia required?

If it does not close on its own by age 4–5 years, causes symptoms (e.g., pain), or becomes incarcerated/ strangulated

True or false: Constipation is defined as decreased frequency of bowel movements.

False. While decreased frequency is often an accompanying symptom, constipation refers to having hard feces, which cause pain and/or are difficult to pass

What is the first-line treatment of constipation?

Increase intake of fluid, bulk food (cereal, vegetables), and pitted fruits and juices

What is a cause of constipation that you do not want to miss in a newborn with delayed passage of meconium or a child with chronic constipation (also abdominal distension, bilious vomiting, failure to thrive)?

Hirschsprung's disease

What is encopresis?

Fecal soiling—often occurs with constipation as looser stool moves around an impaction

What is the most common infectious cause of diarrhea in infants?

Rotavirus

What are the symptoms associated with rotavirus infection?

Watery diarrhea; Fever; Vomiting; Perhaps abdominal pain

What complication do you want to rule out when seeing a patient with diarrhea?

Dehydration

What are the signs of dehydration in an infant?

Elevated heart rate; Lethargy; Poor capillary refill; Skin tenting; Decreased urination; Dry mucous membranes (eyes, oral mucosa)

What is the treatment for mild-to-moderate dehydration secondary to diarrhea?

Oral rehydration therapy (ORT); Avoid sports drinks, sodas, and other sugary items

How do you administer ORT?

50–100 mL/kg over 4 hours initially, then 10 mL/kg for each additional stool

What are some signs of severe dehydration?

Rapid/weak pulses; Decreased blood pressure; No urine output; Very sunken eyes/fontanelles; Dry mucous membranes; Tented or mottled skin; Delayed capillary refill

When are IV fluids required to treat dehydration secondary to diarrhea?

Severe dehydration; Uncontrollable vomiting; Inability to drink because of extreme fatigue or decreased level of consciousness; GI distention

What are some noninfectious causes of diarrhea in children?

Overfeeding; Malabsorption; Necrotizing enterocolitis (NEC); Strangulated hernia; Ovarian/testicular torsion; Mesenteric thrombus

What is intussusception?

Telescoping of one part of small bowel over another

What are the signs and symptoms?

Cramping abdominal pain; Abdominal pain; Vomiting; Blood and mucous in the stool (currant jelly stool)

What is a Meckel's diverticulum?

Outpouching from the small bowel, which has the potential to become inflamed, ulcerate/perforate, or cause bowel obstruction

PULMONOLOGY

What is the most common cause of respiratory failure in premature newborns?

Respiratory distress syndrome

What are the causes of respiratory distress in a newborn?

Respiratory distress syndrome; Transient tachypnea of the newborn; Meconium aspiration; Pneumonia; Heart disease

What are some signs of respiratory distress in an infant/young child?

Tachypnea or bradypnea; Grunting; Cyanosis; Nasal flaring; Retractions and use of accessory muscles

What is the most common chronic lung disease in children?

Asthma

What are the symptoms of asthma in children?

Prolonged expiratory phase with end expiratory wheezes; Typically, *coughing* in younger children, *wheezing* in older children; Chest tightness, dyspnea

Do the symptoms of asthma tend to be worse during the day or at night?

Night

What are some other causes of wheezing?

Anything that restricts the airways: foreign body aspiration; Congenital heart disease; Tracheomalacia; Cystic fibrosis; Bronchiolitis

What are the different classifications of severity of asthma?

Intermittent; Mild persistent (> two symptoms per week); Moderate persistent (daily symptoms); Severe persistent (continuous symptoms)

What is the preventative treatment of asthma?

Long-term low/medium-dose inhaled steroid for mild and moderate persistent types; High-dose inhaled and oral steroids for severe type

What kind of rescue inhaler should be given to all patients with asthma?

Rescue short-acting beta-agonist

What is more efficacious, a beta-agonist administered by inhaler or nebulizer?

Equally efficacious

Should you use mucolytics during an attack?

Contraindicated since they can lead to bronchospasm

What are some causes of viral pneumonia?

Respiratory syncytial virus; Parainfluenza; Adenovirus; Enterovirus

What are some causes of bacterial pneumonia?

Streptococcus pneumonia; Group A *Streptococcus*; Group B *Streptococcus* (in a neonate); *Mycoplasma pneumoniae*; *Chlamydia trachomatis*; *Haemophilus influenza*; *Moraxella catarrhalis*

What is the most common bacterial pneumonia in children less than six years old?

Mycoplasma ("walking pneumonia")

What is the treatment?

Erythromycin or other macrolide antibiotic

What genetic (autosomal recessive) disease causes pancreatic insufficiency and frequent pulmonary infections secondary to mucous plugs?

Cystic fibrosis

NEUROLOGY

Febrile seizures typically occur in what age group?	Six months to five years
Can a febrile seizure cause disability or death?	No
What are the most common bacterial causes of meningitis in the neonatal period?	Group B *Streptococcus; Listeria; Escherichia coli*
In infants more than one month old	*Streptococcus pneumoniae; Neisseria meningitidis*
What are the signs and symptoms of meningitis in an infant?	Decreased appetite; Lethargy; Irritability; Fever; Vomiting; Bulging fontanelle; Seizures
In children	Fever; Lethargy; Photosensitivity; Nausea; Vomiting; Neck stiffness or pain; Headache; Seizures; Positive Kernig's and Brudzinski's signs
What is Kernig's sign?	Inability to extend knee when hips are flexed to 90°
What is Brudzinski's sign?	Passive flexion of the head causes involuntary hip flexion
What is cerebral palsy (CP)?	A nonprogressive movement disorder associated with perinatal brain damage
Is CP hereditary?	No

INFECTIOUS DISEASE

What is croup?	Acute laryngotracheitis
What is the most common cause?	Parainfluenza virus
What is the radiographic finding known as the "steeple sign"?	Anteroposterior (AP) view of the neck shows narrowing trachea
What is the treatment?	Steroids, nebulizer treatments, cool humidified air; Hospitalization for toxic-appearing children
What is the infectious agent of pertussis (whooping cough)?	*Bordetella pertussis*

What are the classic symptoms?	Whooping coughing spells (paroxysms) followed by post-tussive emesis
What are the three stages of disease?	1. Catarrhal stage (mild upper respiratory infection (URI) symptoms) 2. Paroxysmal (whooping cough) 3. Convalescent (mild cough continues)
How long may it last?	12 weeks
Do antibiotics abort the disease?	Only in the catarrhal phase
So why give antibiotics?	To decrease spread to others
What is the drug of choice?	Erythromycin
What is the concerning possible complication of erythromycin in infants?	Hypertrophic pyloric stenosis
What are alternatives to erythromycin?	Other macrolides (e.g., azithromycin)

Answer the following questions about sinus development and sinusitis in children.

Name the four sinus cavities.	1. Ethmoid 2. Maxillary 3. Frontal 4. Sphenoid
Which of these are present at birth?	Ethmoid; Maxillary
Which begins development at age two years but is only apparent by x-ray until five years?	Sphenoid
Which is the last to develop?	Frontal (starts developing at age four years and may grow up until 20)
Why is the order of sinus development important?	In children, most infections involve the ethmoid and maxillary sinuses; and frontal and sphenoid infections usually begin to appear in adolescence
True or false: Children with sinusitis often complain of headache and facial pain.	False. Remember the location of the earlier developing sinuses
What is an exanthem?	The cutaneous manifestation of an infectious disease

Name the infectious agent of the following six classic exanthems:

Measles	Measles virus
Rubella	Rubella virus
Erythema infectiosum (i.e., Fifth disease)	Parvovirus B19
Roseola	Human herpesvirus 6 (HHV6)
Varicella	Varicella-zoster virus
Scarlet fever	*Streptococcus pyogenes*

With regards to measles:

What is the first sign?	Koplik's spots—white papules on red base on the buccal surfaces
Describe the rash.	Erythematous maculopapular; Progresses cephalocaudally; Regresses cephalocaudally
What are the worrisome complications?	Pneumonia; Encephalitis; Subacute sclerosing panencephalitis

With regards to rubella:

Describe the rash.	Fleeting, discreet macules
When is it particularly dangerous and why?	Infection in pregnant women causes embryopathy

With regards to roseola:

Describe the natural course.	High fever for three days; then rash appears when fever drops
What is the progression of the rash?	Starts on the trunk and spreads to the extremities
What is the treatment?	Supportive
What is the classic rash of Fifth disease?	Slapped cheeks and lacy rash (trunk→arms and legs)
What is the classic rash of varicella?	Crops of vesicles (dew drops on a red base) beginning on trunk

MISCELLANEOUS

What etiology should you suspect in a child with recurrent urinary tract infections (UTIs)?	Vesicoureteral reflux

What test do you order to evaluate for vesicoureteral reflux?	Voiding cystourethrogram
What is the most common cause of nephrotic syndrome in children?	Minimal change disease
What is the treatment?	Steroids
What is the most common cause of anemia in children?	Iron deficiency
What is the most common childhood malignancy?	Leukemia
What is the usual initial presentation of leukemia?	Vague symptoms such as weight loss, anorexia, and fatigue

CHAPTER 18

Clinical Vignettes

A young adult male complains of fever for 1 week, joint pain, and a sore throat (despite ibuprofen and throat lozenges). He had unprotected sex 3 weeks ago. Examination: T 38°C, cervical lymphadenopathy, supple neck, faint macular rash, pharyngitis with exudates.

What tests do you order?

Complete blood count (CBC); Monospot test; Throat culture (include testing for gonorrhea and chlamydia); HIV viral load by polymerase chain reaction (PCR)

If you suspect HIV infection why not order enzyme-linked immunosorbent assay (ELISA) and Western blot tests?

They can be negative in the acute phase

What vaccines should you give this patient?

Tetanus; Pneumococcus; Hepatitis A and B (if serology is negative); Intramuscular influenza (depending on time of year)

A plasma HIV-RNA viral load can be used for what reasons?

To assess a baseline viral load; To assess drug efficacy; To help decide when to begin anti-viral therapy; To guide changes in prophylactic therapy (PCP, MAC, etc.)

A 56-year-old male comes to your clinic for a physical examination and you give him a clean bill of health. He is normotensive.

Knowing nothing else about his history and physical, what is this patient's lifetime risk of developing hypertension (HTN)

According to JNC7, normotensive adults over 50 years have a 90% lifetime risk of developing HTN

A few years later the same pt comes back, is overweight, and his blood pressure (BP) is 135/85. The rest of the

Prehypertension

examination is normal. What is your diagnosis? Assume that you subsequently confirm the BP.

What lifestyle modifications would you recommend?

Weight reduction; Dietary approaches to stop hypertension (DASH) diet; Physical activity; No more than 1 oz of alcohol per day

If this patient later develops hypertension, but has no other comorbidities, what would be your first line of drug therapy?

Thiazide diuretic

A healthy-appearing 65-year-old male comes in for his yearly examination. He wears reading glasses (review of systems is otherwise negative). He is retired, eats well, and plays tennis three times a week with his wife. Body mass index (BMI) = 23.5 kg/m^2

His last colonoscopy (at age 60) showed no abnormalities. Assuming he remains asymptomatic, when should he repeat colon cancer screening?

70 years

For what other diseases would you screen this patient? (Level A and B recommendations by US Preventive Services Task Force [USPSTF])

Level A: Hyperlipidemia; HTN
Level B: Alcohol misuse; Depression; Diabetes mellitus (DM) Type II (if patient turns out to have hyperlipidemia or HTN)

Would you screen for prostate cancer?

Maybe. There is insufficient evidence recommending for or against screening. Have an individualized discussion with your patient regarding this screening before making a decision

If he tells you he smoked one pack of cigarettes a week for one year when he was in his forties, what other screening(s) would you do?

Screen for abdominal aortic aneurysm with abdominal ultrasonography

What are the recommended immunizations for this patient?

Tetanus; Pneumococcal; Influenza

A ten-month old is febrile and irritable. He did not sleep well last night and has been pulling on his right ear. Mom says, "He is getting over a cold." Examination: Right tympanic membrane is bulging and immobile.

What is the most likely diagnosis?

Acute otitis media

What is your treatment?

Pain medication (ibuprofen or acetaminophen); Amoxicillin (although some advocate a "wait and see" approach vs. antibiotics)

He comes back at his one-year well-child visit. His mom says that he has been "healthy and happy." You note air bubbles behind the Tympanic membrane (TM) and the rest of his examination is normal. What is your diagnosis?

Otitis media with effusion

What do you do?

Schedule follow-up visit and perhaps a hearing test, but do not prescribe antibiotics

12 weeks after the initial AOM, the patient still has the effusion. Now what?

Order hearing test if you have not already and refer to ENT (may need ear tubes)

A 48-year-old obese female comes into the office stating that her right hip has been hurting for a couple of weeks and she cannot sleep on her right side. The rest of her review of systems is noncontributory. Examination: Point tenderness over the greater trochanter, but otherwise normal.

What is the most likely initial diagnosis?

Non-septic trochanteric bursitis

What physical examination findings could be indicative of a more serious condition?

Skin changes; Fever; Other signs of infection

Where is the hip joint located, and is this patient truly experiencing "hip pain?"

The hip joints (which are affected in diseases like osteoarthritis) attach to the pelvis in the *groin*. Her pain is over the greater trochanter bursa along the lateral thigh. This is important to note because patients will often complain of "hip pain" with bursitis and "groin pain" with OA

Assuming that you decide to treat the patient with a corticosteroid shot, is aspiration prior to the shot indicated, and if so, why?

No. While it is a good idea to aspirate superficial bursa with obvious swelling and/or infection, aspiration at deep bursae yield little to no fluid and only causes patient discomfort

A 65-year-old female complains of
a seven-month history of knee pain and
stiffness, worse at the end of the day. She
has also been noticing pain in her hips,
back, and hands, particularly at the base
of the thumbs.

What is the most likely diagnosis?	Osteoarthritis
You notice a square appearance of the radial aspect of her hands. What is this finding called?	Shelf sign
What is the most *specific* radiographic marker for OA?	Osteophytes
Why is exercise important for this patient?	Exercise prevents muscle spasm and atrophy, helps to keep down body weight, and improves other aspects of general health
What kind would you recommend?	Care should be taken to minimize weight-bearing exercises (swimming is ideal) in order to not accelerate the need for surgery

A 30-year-old female complains of severe
and episodic left-sided throbbing
headache that lasts 4 hours. Sleeping in
a dark and quiet room helps relieve her
symptoms. ROS: nausea/vomiting with
headache. FH: Mother and sister have
had similar symptoms. Examination:
normal.

What is the *most likely* diagnosis?	Migraine headache
Assuming the most likely diagnosis is correct, under what circumstances would you consider prophylactic treatment for this patient?	Three or more headaches a month; Headaches occur at predictable times (e.g., menses); Acute therapy is not effective; The headaches cause severe symptoms (e.g., hemiplegia) and/or the patient feels debilitated
What medications are used for prophylactic treatment?	Beta-blockers; Anti-seizure medications; Calcium-channel blockers; Tricyclic antidepressants
What medications are used for acute (abortive) treatment?	Serotonin agonists (i.e., triptans); Ergotamine; Nonsteroid anti-inflammatory drugs (NSAIDs) Occasionally narcotic pain meds

What kind of radiographic testing does this patient need?	Testing is unnecessary for most young and otherwise healthy patients presenting with headache (unless there are localizing neurologic symptoms or signs of intracranial hypertension)

A 65-year-old male complains of chest pain.

What are your highest diagnostic priorities?	Distinguishing cardiac from non-cardiac and life-threatening from non-emergent causes of chest pain
He says the pain has a squeezing quality and radiates to his jaw. Episodes last two minutes, are brought on by exercise, and relieved with rest. The pain is not associated with food intake, and not relieved by antacids. He denies fever, diaphoresis, dyspnea, and nausea. What is the *most likely* diagnosis?	Stable angina resulting from ischemic heart disease
What tests help you rule out an myocardial infarction (MI)?	Cardiac enzymes; ECG
Assuming that the MI workup is negative, what noninvasive test would you use to assess the degree of ischemic heart disease?	Exercise stress test (assuming that the patient can tolerate it)
What medications are available to treat anginal pain?	Nitrates; Beta-blockers; Calcium-channel blockers

A 50-year-old male with a history of type II diabetes mellitus and hypertension presents to your office for a well-man examination.

What is his goal BP?	Systolic blood pressure <130 and diastolic blood pressure <80
His BP is 145/73, and his BP on the previous visit was 132/78. Which anti-hypertensive should be started?	An angiotensin-converting enzyme (ACE) inhibitor
Being a conscientious doctor, you order a fasting lipid panel. Low-density lipoprotein (LDL) is 140. What should you do next?	Start a statin. As a diabetic, his LDL goal is less than 100

A 45-year-old male with a history of
hypertension presents with acute onset of
right knee pain and swelling.

What is the differential diagnosis?

Gout; Pseudogout; Acute septic
arthritis; Bacterial cellulitis;
Traumatic injury to joint

Knowing that he was recently started
on hydrochlorothiazide for better BP
control increases the possibility
of which diagnosis?

Gout

If you order a uric acid level and it is
normal, does this rule out gout?

No. The level may be falsely low
during an acute attack

Your working diagnosis is an acute
gouty attack. How do you confirm your
diagnosis?

Aspiration of the synovial fluid with
visualization of negatively
birefringent, needle-shaped crystals

Two months later, he returns to your
office and complains of flank pain.
What diagnosis should be on your
differential?

Uric acid nephrolithiasis

A young adult female presents with
a 3-week history of bilateral wrist pain.
On review of systems, she has only
noticed mild gum bleeding and mild
fatigue. Electrolytes are normal. WBC is
2.1, platelets are 109, and hemoglobin
is 10.5.

Given her arthritis and pancytopenia,
you want to rule out systemic lupus
erythematous. What tests should you
order?

Antinuclear antibody (ANA); Anti-
dsDNA; Anti-Smith antibodies

Which of the immunologic tests best
correlates with lupus flares?

Anti-dsDNA antibodies

She later presents to your office with
a blood pressure of 142/80. Which
studies should you order?

Creatinine; Urinalysis;
24-hour urine protein to evaluate
nephropathy secondary to lupus

A 56-year-old woman presents to your
office for a well-woman examination. She
had a normal double-contrast barium
enema at age 50, a normal Pap smear at
age 54, and a normal mammogram at
age 52.

She has been in a monogamous
relationship for 30 years. If she has

No. With normal Pap smears, she
can get a Pap smear every 2–3 years

always had normal Pap smears, does
she need a Pap smear this year?

Does she need colon cancer screening this year?	Yes
Is she due for a mammogram this year?	Yes. She should receive a mammogram every 1–2 years

A 32-year-old G1P0 woman at 32-weeks
gestational age presents for a routine visit.
Looking through her labs, you notice that
she is rubella nonimmune and HBsAg
positive.

Should you administer the rubella vaccine at this visit?	No. Live vaccines should not be given to pregnant women (wait until she is postpartum)
What treatment should you provide to the baby at birth?	Hepatitis B immunoglobulin; The first dose of the hepatitis B vaccine
Which vaccines should you provide at the baby's two-month visit?	DTaP; Hib; IPV; PCV7 (may give the second hepatitis B)

A 35-year-old woman with a history of
lupus, well-controlled with methotrexate,
presents to your office with a two-month
history of fatigue. She saw another doctor
one month ago and was given FeSO4
(325 mg PO daily).

After the history and physical, what is the first step in your workup?	Check a CBC to confirm the diagnosis of anemia
Hemoglobin is 9.6, and the mean corpuscular volume (MCV) is 101. Is her anemia likely due to iron deficiency?	No
Based on the MCV, can you rule out iron deficiency anemia?	No. Two kinds of anemia can be present simultaneously and the MCV is an average value
What studies help you rule out iron deficiency?	Serum iron, ferritin, transferrin, total iron-binding capacity (TIBC)
Her iron studies are normal, so you know she has strictly macrocytic anemia. What is the differential diagnosis?	Folate deficiency; Vitamin B_{12} deficiency; Certain drugs (hydroxyurea and AZT); Liver disease; Hypothyroidism; Hyperlipidemia; Alcohol abuse; Myelodysplastic disorders
What is the most likely cause of her macrocytic anemia?	Folate deficiency secondary to methotrexate

A 55-year-old woman s/p recent right knee replacement presents with right calf tenderness.

You suspect a deep vein thrombosis (DVT), and the D-dimer is 561. Should you start anticoagulation?	No. D-dimer has a high negative predictive value. D-dimer greater than 500 does not confirm a diagnosis of DVT
What should you order to diagnose a DVT?	Compression ultrasonography
Ultrasonography reveals a deep venous thrombosis. What medication should you start?	Start unfractionated heparin (UFH) or low molecular-weight heparin (LMWH) initially; Coumadin for long-term treatment
If she also has severe renal insufficiency, would you choose UFH or LMWH?	Use UFH, since LMWH is excreted mainly by the kidneys
What international normalized ratio (INR) is therapeutic for this patient?	2–3
Two months later, she presents to your office with left-sided chest pain. Having run out of coumadin, the patient's INR is 1.2. Her ECG is normal except for sinus tachycardia. What diagnosis should you consider and how would you confirm the diagnosis?	Pulmonary embolism. Diagnose with a V/Q scan, spiral CT, or pulmonary angiography

A 19-year-old woman with a 5-pack-year history of smoking presents to your office for a well-woman examination. She has been sexually active since age 16 and has had multiple partners.

Does she need a Pap smear?	Yes. The initial Pap smear should be at age 21 or 3 years after first starting intercourse, whichever comes first
The Pap smear comes back ASCUS (i.e., a typical squamous cells of undetermined significance) and is positive for high-risk human papillomavirus (HPV) serotypes. What test should you order next?	Colposcopy
Colposcopy is negative for malignancy. What is the next step in the management of this patient?	Repeat a Pap smear with reflex HPV testing in 12 months

A 21-year-old woman presents to your office with a four-day history of profuse vaginal discharge.

What is the next step in the workup of vaginal discharge?	KOH and saline mounts
You suspect trichomonas. What would you see on a saline mount of the discharge?	Motile, flagellated trichomonads

The pH of the discharge is 5.5. Is this consistent with a diagnosis of trichomonas?

Yes. The pH is elevated (>4.5)

Besides prescribing the patient with metronidazole, what else should you do?	Treat her partner too

A 45-year-old healthy woman says she awoke with a "red eye." She denies pain or history of trauma. Examination: well-circumscribed portion of the eye is completely red without evidence of conjunctival inflammation. Vision is normal.

What is the most likely diagnosis?	Subconjunctival hemorrhage
What are the underlying causes of subconjunctival hemorrhages?	Subconjunctival hemorrhages may occur spontaneously or secondary to trauma
What is the appropriate management of a subconjunctival hemorrhage?	They usually spontaneously clear within 2–3 weeks, so no treatment is necessary
What should be considered if a patient experiences repeated subconjunctival hemorrhages?	Workup for a bleeding disorder

A 65-year-old presents with a vague history of joint pain, weight loss, scalp tenderness, and a unilateral headache associated with pain in the jaw when chewing.

What is the most likely diagnosis?	Giant cell arteritis (GCA) (i.e., temporal arteritis)
What workup helps you make the diagnosis?	Careful physical examination for tender arteries or bruits; Elevated erythrocyte sedimentation rate (ESR) or c-reactive protein (CRP); Temporal artery biopsy
Patients with GCA are at increased risk for what ocular problems?	Ischemic optic neuropathy; Central retinal artery occlusion; Paresis of extraocular movements

What is the mandatory treatment of GCA?	High-dose oral corticosteroids unless there is a strong contraindication. Start treatment ASAP (do not need to wait for result of biopsy).

A 70-year-old male presents complaining of "forgetfulness" (gradual onset over the past months). His wife has noticed changes in his memory for more than a year and says he has become more withdrawn, although the patient denies this. A depression screen is negative.

What is the most likely diagnosis?	Dementia
What percentage of patients have a potentially reversible form of dementia?	15%
What minimum lab workup should you do to determine if the condition is reversible?	CBC; Electrolytes; TFTs; VDRL/RPR; HIV; B_{12}/Folate; Brain CT or MRI
If the patient also complained of urinary incontinence, ataxia or had dilated cerebral ventricles on imaging, what is the most likely diagnosis ?	Normal pressure hydrocephalus
If all the tests are within normal limits, except for diffuse atrophy and flattened sulci on imaging, what is the most likely diagnosis?	Alzheimer's disease
What class of drugs can help slow the progression of Alzheimer's disease?	Cholinesterase inhibitors (Donepezil, Rivastigmine); NMDA receptor antagonist (Namenda)

A 23-year-old G2 now P2 s/p Day #2 from a repeat c-section has a firm but tender fundus on examination. She also has fever, tachycardia, and foul-smelling lochia.

What is the most likely diagnosis?	Endomyometritis
What are other common causes of post-op fever?	Wound infection; Atelectasis; Urinary tract infection; DVT; Drug fever
What kind of antibiotics would you use to treat her presumed endomyometritis?	Clindamycin plus an aminoglycoside (such as gentamicin)
Why do you need clindamycin?	Anaerobic coverage (she is s/p c-section)

A 65-year-old male needs surgical clearance for a prostatectomy. He has a ten-year history of HTN and has a carotid bruit on

examination. The rest of the H&P is
noncontributory.

> **What are the general goals of surgical
> clearance?**

Assess the severity of disease; Decide
if a patient can tolerate surgery; If so,
optimize treatment before surgery

> **What cardiovascular studies would you
> obtain before clearing this patient?**

ECG; Carotid dopplers

> **If he is on aspirin, how long before the
> surgery should he stop taking it?**

A week before surgery

> **He is on both a beta-blocker and
> thiazide diuretic. Which should he
> hold the day of surgery and why?**

Hold the diuretic. The patient is
already NPO and further diuresis
could cause severe hypovolemia

A 25-year-old male presents for a new
patient physical. On examination, you
notice a painless enlargement of one of
his testes. He has no other symptoms.

> **What is the most likely diagnosis?**

Testicular cancer

> **What are the most common symptoms
> of testicular tumor?**

No symptoms (80%) or symptoms of
epididymitis (15–20%)

> **Testicular cancer is most prevalent in
> what age group?**

15–35-year olds

> **How is the diagnosis made (including
> staging)?**

Testicular ultrasound; CXR and
abdominal pelvic CT for mets;
B-hCG; Alpha-fetoprotein

> **What percentage of testicular tumors
> are malignant?**

95% (most common malignancy in
men 25–34-years old)

> **What are the risk factors for the
> development of testicular cancer?**

Cryptorchidism and Klinefelter's
syndrome

> **What is the name for an undescended
> testicle?**

Cryptorchidism

> **What testicular malignancy develops
> most commonly later in life in a patient
> with a history of cryptorchidism?**

Seminoma

> **Does surgical correction of the
> undescended testicle decrease the risk
> of malignancy later in life?**

No. But it does allow early detection

A 15-year-old presents to your office with
a worm-like mass in his left scrotum for
a couple of months. He has no other
symptoms, and on examination, the mass
does not involve the testicle.

What is the most likely diagnosis?	Varicocele
What veins swell to form the varicocele?	Pampiniform plexus
What percentage of men evaluated for infertility are found to have a varicocele?	25–30%
On what side do varicoceles most commonly occur?	Left
What physical examination maneuver can make the varicocele enlarge?	Valsalva
If the mass transilluminated, what diagnosis would you suspect?	Hydrocele
What is the treatment of varicocele?	Surgical repair is indicated in an adolescent only if the testicle on the affected side is smaller than the other by 0.5 cm or more

A 20-year-old male presents with an acute, painful swelling of the testicle, with fever, dysuria, and tender scrotal mass on examination.

What is the most likely diagnosis?	Acute epididymitis
What organisms are most commonly responsible for epididymitis in a young male?	*Chlamydia trachomatis; Neisseria gonorrhea*
In an older male	*Escherichia coli* or other coliform bacteria

A 10-year-old presents to the emergency department with acute testicular pain and nausea. On examination, his abdomen is non-tender, but his testicle is tender and retracted. You suspect testicular torsion.

What do you do?	This is a surgical emergency! A testicular scintillation scan confirms the diagnosis (90% specific)

A 67-year-old presents with fever, productive cough, dyspnea, and pleuritic chest pain worsening over 1 week. She is tachypneic, but her breath sounds are clear.

True or false: Clear breath sounds are a good indication that this patient is stable.	False. Her breaths may be too shallow and fast to appreciate adventitious breath sounds

Her chest x-ray shows a right lower lobe consolidation. What is your diagnosis?	Pneumonia
A gram stain of her sputum shows gram-positive diplococci. What kind of antibiotic would you treat her with?	Cephalosporin or fluoroquinolone

A 16-year-old complains of pimples on her face. She has no other medical problems and is not on any medications. Examination: Scattered maculopapular-pustular lesions as well as comedones on her face and back.

What is the most likely diagnosis?	Acne vulgaris
What age group is most affected by this problem?	Teens. But some cases persist through the twenties and thirties
What bacterium is associated with this disorder?	*Propionibacterium acnes*
What is the first-line treatment for this condition?	Topical benzoyl peroxide 2.5% applied twice daily, increasing to 5%, and then 10%. Topical tretinoin or Adapalene can be applied at bedtime
What agents can be added if the above regimen does not resolve the condition?	Topical erythromycin or clindamycin, plus or minus a systemic tetracycline
If the patient presented with severe cystic acne, what treatment option would you consider?	Oral retinoid such as Accutane
What are the absolute contraindications to the use of 13-cis-retinoic acid?	Child under the age of 14; Women of childbearing potential who are not protected against pregnancy (teratogenic to fetus); Allergy to a topical tretinoin
This patient is overweight, has missed several periods, and has noticed excess hair growth. Her pregnancy test is negative. What diagnosis do you suspect?	Polycystic ovarian syndrome (PCOS)
What medication would benefit her if these were the diagnoses?	Oral contraceptives to improve acne and restore menstrual cycles

A 40-year-old man presents to your office complaining of four days of lower back pain after he was moving boxes in his attic. Examination: Normal motor and sensory function, negative straight leg-raise test.

What is the most likely diagnosis?	Lower back strain
Are any diagnostic tests necessary to make the above diagnosis?	No
What is the treatment for lower back strain?	NSAIDs for one week; Supportive modalities such as heat and stretching
If on examination, the patient were found to have decreased sensation in his foot and inability to toe-walk on the right, what would you be concerned about?	Lumbar disc herniation
What is the name for the above symptoms caused by the lumbar disc herniation?	Sciatica
Lumbar disc herniations occur most commonly at what two vertebral levels?	L4–L5 and L5-S1
What percentage of herniated discs spontaneously resorb and do not require surgery?	90–95%
Bladder dysfunction, discrete sensory level, bilateral weakness, and anal sphincter weakness secondary to a centrally herniating lumbar disc is known as what syndrome?	Cauda equina syndrome (requires urgent neurosurgical or orthopedic evaluation)

A seven-month old presents with a two-day history of cough, nasal congestion, and fever (100°F). He has six wet diapers a day and is playful. Examination: Normal except for nasal congestion.

What is the diagnosis?	Upper respiratory tract infection
The patient's mother wants you to prescribe antibiotics. What do you do?	Do not prescribe antibiotics since this is most likely a viral etiology. This is a good opportunity for parent education
He is not up to date on his vaccinations. Is it safe to administer some on this visit?	Yes

A 30-year-old usually healthy female has just returned from her honeymoon and complains of urinary frequency and dysuria for two days. She is otherwise healthy and takes OCPs.

What is the most likely diagnosis?	Urinary tract infection
A urinalysis (UA) shows positive leukocyte esterase and nitrite. How do you treat this patient?	Trimethoprim/sulfamethoxazole double-strength tablet PO daily for three days (watch for resistance—may need a fluoroquinolone)
What recommendations would you make to decrease her risk of urinary tract infections in the future?	Drink plenty of fluids; Void after intercourse; Wipe from front to back; Avoid using deodorant sprays; Other potentially irritating feminine products (douches, powders)

A 6-year-old usually healthy boy presents with a sore throat and fever (102.5°F) but no cough or nasal congestion. Examination: Tender cervical lymphadenopathy, tonsillar erythema, and exudates.

What is the most likely diagnosis?	Pharyngitis
What is the most likely etiologic agent?	A virus or Streptococcus
What is the only cause of pharyngitis that requires antibiotic treatment?	Group A beta-hemolytic Streptococcus
How would you go about diagnosing strep throat?	Streptococcal antigen testing ("rapid strep test")
Your test comes back positive, how would you treat this patient?	Oral penicillin V potassium for ten days
His mom says she does not feel like she can "make him take antibiotics for ten days." What is an alternative treatment?	One time dose of penicillin G benzathine IM
What antibiotics are alternatives if the patient is allergic to penicillin?	Erythromycin or azithromycin

A 50-year-old male with a history of lower back strain (for which he takes ibuprofen) complains of "burning" abdominal pain and melena, but does not complain of vomiting or constipation.

What is the most likely diagnosis?	Gastrointestinal (GI) bleeding secondary to NSAID-induced ulcer or gastritis
Why is checking his vitals, including orthostatics, so important?	To assess the patient's hemodynamic and fluid status (hypovolemia)
On examination, you notice signs of portal hypertension, and he admits to	Esophageal varices

heavy alcohol use. What would you
add to your differential?

Once the patient is stable, what test   Esophagogastroduodenoscopy
would you order to evaluate (possibly   (EGD)
treat) the source of bleeding?

Index